From an Association to a Royal College

Alan Craft · Keith Dodd

Editors

From an Association to a Royal College

The History of the British Paediatric Association and Royal College of Paediatrics and Child Health 1988–2016

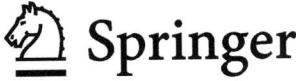 Springer

Editors
Alan Craft
Sir James Spence Institute
Newcastle University
Newcastle upon Tyne
UK

Keith Dodd
Derbyshire Children's Hospital
Derby
UK

ISBN 978-3-319-43581-7   ISBN 978-3-319-43582-4   (eBook)
DOI 10.1007/978-3-319-43582-4

Library of Congress Control Number: 2016958530

Printed on acid-free paper

This Springer imprint is published by Springer Nature
The registered company is Springer International Publishing AG
The registered company address is Gewerbestrasse 11, 6330 Cham, Switzerland

The health of infants, children and young people is at the core of all we do

The RCPCH aims to ensure every paediatrician has the knowledge and expertise to promote child health and to care for infants, children and young people with health needs

The RCPCH aims to improve the health and wellbeing on infants, children and young people in the UK and across the developing world

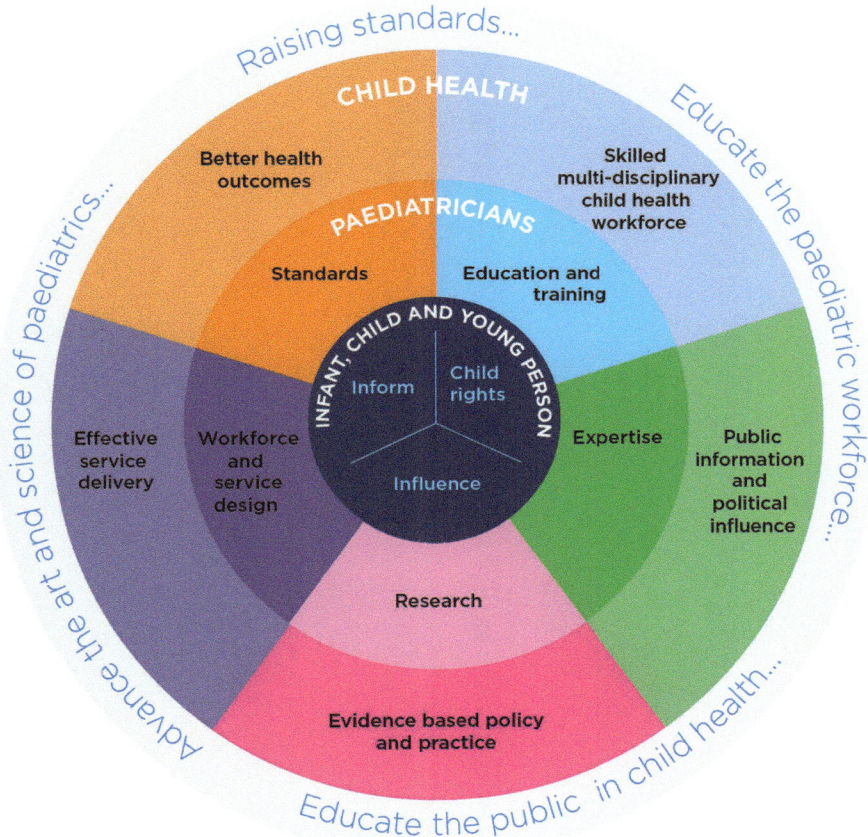

Foreword

Her Royal Highness Princess Anne, Patron of the RCPCH

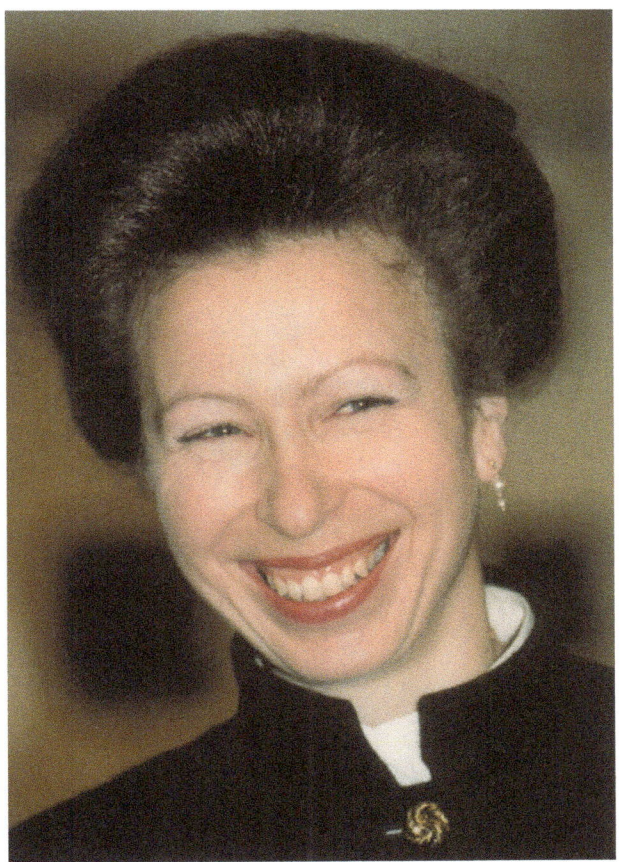

Buckingham Palace

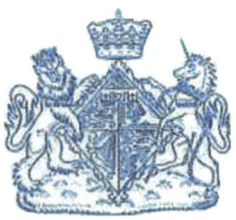

As the Royal College of Paediatrics and Child Health (RCPCH) approaches its 21st birthday, I am delighted to write the foreword for this history book. The Royal Charter was granted in 1996, and I have been the Patron of the College since that year. I have been pleased to see the charity grow in size and influence over the years. The book provides many insightful and personal reflections. It includes descriptions of the problems overcome as the College strove, in the early days, to achieve true independence and recognition for its role as educators of paediatricians. The authors reinforce the additional unique overarching focus of the RCPCH as a College concerned with the high-quality care of sick children and the improvement of child health, not only in the UK but worldwide.

The book provides personal accounts of its activity to ensure evidence-based paediatric practice and service standards and its role in informing policymakers and for providing education of not only all health professionals working with children but also the public. Children and young people are discussed as true partners in the activity of the RCPCH, directing areas for development, and indeed their presence and engagement have been evident at recent RCPCH events I have had the pleasure to attend. What comes across throughout this book is 21 years of dedication and commitment to improving health outcomes for the youngest in our society.

Anne

Introduction

In 1928, the five men who met in Dr Still's house in Queen Anne Street, London, to form the British Paediatric Association (BPA) could not have envisaged where that fledgling organisation would be almost 90 years later. They sent out invitations to 24 men who were beginning to develop the specialty of paediatrics and most accepted. The first aim was to bring together like-minded people who shared a common interest in caring for children, but they had no reason to meet together other than a bond of friendship.

Throughout the last 90 years, there have been three official records of the progress which has been made, with Hector Cameron recording 1928–1952, Victor Neale the period from 1952 to 1968 and John Forfar, Tony Jackson and Bernard Laurence bringing us up to 1988.

A special volume was produced by Bernard Valman at the millennium which chronicled something of the transition from a professional association to a Royal College. We, as the editors of this latest volume, have had the privilege to serve as officers through this momentous period in our history. We have gone from the original 18 members in 1928 to over 16,000 in 2015. We have grown from a friendly club who met to share a common interest to one which now sets and maintains the standards of the training for doctors who want to work with children and also influences the way that services are delivered.

Most of today's members have joined in the last 20 years and will have little idea of our roots and of the journey on which we have come to be an independent voice for children and those doctors who care for them.

We have therefore included as an appendix an extract from the third volume of the BPA history which chronicles the efforts from 1928 to 1987 of the real pioneers in children's health. The first President of the Royal College of Paediatrics and Child Health (RCPCH), Professor Sir Roy Meadow, wrote what is generally accepted to be a good, fair and accurate account of the struggle to make the giant step to a Royal College, and we reproduce it here from the *Millennium* book. There were many sides to the story of eventually becoming a College, and the debates often became heated and, at times, acrimonious. We have asked several of the key players of the time to reflect on their roles and to address the question as to whether the struggle was worthwhile.

As will be seen, the major issue was not so much whether there should be a separate College of Paediatrics, but rather that creating yet another Medical Royal

College would dilute the traditional influence and power of the ancient Colleges of Physicians and Surgeons who had built their power bases over centuries, to be joined by the pathologists, the obstetricians and a string of smaller specialties.

There is little doubt that the advent of the NHS in 1947 made health care overtly political and successive governments have flexed their muscles to get or retain control of what is now a £120 billion budget. The government has to relate to the British Medical Association (BMA) as the doctors' trade union, but the collective Royal Colleges retain an important role in setting and maintaining professional standards and giving advice on health and related matters.

The RCPCH may be one of the youngest of the Royal Colleges but is by no means the smallest or least influential.

In this volume, we have asked contributors to reflect on different aspects of the College's work. It cannot be a complete record of everything the College and its members are now engaged in nor of the breadth of its influence. But we hope that it will be read as a record of where we are, and where we have come from, and that it will be a stepping stone to the centenary history in 2028.

We are enormously grateful to all of our contributors and to Professor Judith Ellis and her staff at the RCPCH.

Professor Sir Alan Craft and Dr Keith Dodd

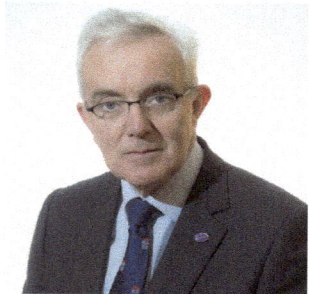

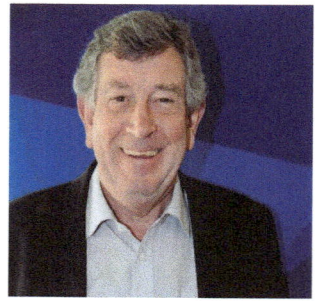

Alan Craft
Newcastle upon Tyne, UK

Keith Dodd
Derby, UK

Contents

Winning the Battle for a College

Roy Meadow

The previous histories *The British Paediatric Association 1928–1988* (see Appendix) reveals how the topic of college status became an increasingly important subject of discussion and debate for paediatricians. During the 1970s and 1980s, the subject dominated the business at annual general meetings (AGMs) and led to important referenda of BPA members.

The 1987 referendum had shown almost equal support for a Faculty of Paediatrics within the Royal Colleges of Physicians (RCPs) of the UK and an independent college. The outgoing president, John Forfar, and his successor, June Lloyd, were members of a subcommittee established to consider the result of that referendum. It

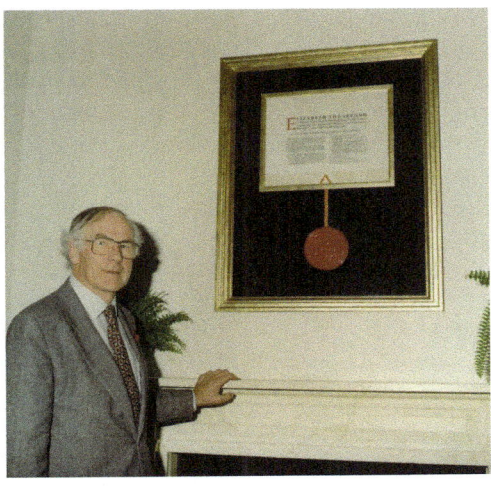

Professor Sir Roy Meadow with the Royal Charter

R. Meadow
Leeds, UK

© Springer International Publishing Switzerland 2017
A. Craft, K. Dodd (eds.), *From an Association to a Royal College*,
DOI 10.1007/978-3-319-43582-4_1

proposed to council that steps should be taken to establish a college of paediatricians *interdependent* with the three RCPs. With council's support, the motion was overwhelmingly accepted at the 1988 AGM in York.

However, much depended upon the interpretation of *interdependent*. Difficult negotiations commenced with the London, Edinburgh and Glasgow Colleges. The outcome was a series of proposals which were put to BPA members in 1990 and which culminated in a referendum on the question 'should the British Paediatric Association proceed to establish closer integration with the Royal Colleges of Physicians of the UK, as outlined in the attached proposals, but continue to maintain its independence to speak on behalf of paediatrics and child health?' In the subsequent ballot, 469 (38.5%) voted 'yes' and 745 (61.5%) voted 'no'. Thus, proposals to integrate the BPA more closely with the RCPs were doomed. The corollary was that those who favoured an independent college believed that the wind of change was strengthening and that the many new colleagues in the rapidly expanding specialty of paediatrics felt less allegiance to the RCPs than did their predecessors.

More than half of the BPA's 2,400 members had joined in the previous 10 years, and their training and life had changed dramatically in that time. Unlike their teachers, trainees were entering paediatrics immediately after registration. In the past, most paediatricians had had to work in adult medicine in order to pass the adult MRCP, but the creation of a paediatric MRCP Clinical Examination altered that. Moreover, it was clear that European law was going to demand a more structured and shorter specialist training, which would entail total immersion in paediatrics.

June Lloyd, the president, though personally committed to an independent college, had represented the divergence of views within the association with great integrity and had conducted the negotiations with the three RCPs with care and firmness. The 1990 vote, however, was a signal that paediatricians might be prepared to commit themselves to change. The incoming president was David Hull. He had been elected unopposed and commanded great respect. In the past, he had been a listener rather than a mover in the debates about college status. However, in his first year of presidency, he quickly demonstrated his commitment to change by leading the council to seek a further referendum of members, in March 1992, to answer the question 'do you wish the British Paediatric Association to proceed to apply for a charter to become a college?' Of 1,267 ballot papers returned, 62% were in favour, and 38% were against. Some of those disagreeing with the outcome pointed out that 700 members had not taken up the opportunity to vote and, therefore, there was not a clear majority in favour of college status. Most members, though, accepted that the referendum result was a mandate for change and the council and its officers were clear in that view. Following a unanimous vote of BPA Council in June 1992, the honorary officers were instructed to proceed to seek a charter to become a college.

Negotiations with the Privy Council

Detailed planning began. To become a college, the BPA had to lodge its application with the Privy Council. Mr Bertie Leigh, of Hempsons Solicitors, was engaged to draft the petition, bye-laws and charter. Preliminary meetings were held between senior officers of the Privy Council and senior BPA officers. The meetings took place in the Cabinet Office at the corner of Downing Street and Whitehall. Those of us participating were met with courtesy (and cups of tea). The main impression from the meetings with the Privy Council officers was of their caution, their reluctance to consider change, their respect for the ancient Colleges and their wish not to upset the status quo. At one of the early meetings, the clerk to the Privy Council asked if the BPA had considered the possibility of becoming a Faculty of the RCP! Despite the negative vibrations, the BPA officers and secretariat worked with Hempsons to produce the draft petition, bye-laws and charter. These were approved by the BPA Council before being lodged formally with the Privy Council in February 1994. The draft petition required a resolution to be put to our AGM. At the April 1994 AGM in Warwick, the last to be presided over by David Hull, members voted by an overwhelming majority (94 %) in favour of empowering the council of the association 'to take all the necessary steps to petition the Queen's most Excellent Majesty and Council'.

In the *London Gazette* of 22 July 1994, notice was given of the petition from the BPA, asking that all petitions for or against the granting of a royal charter should be delivered to the Privy Council before 13 September 1994.

During the final 6 months of his presidency, David Hull had taken time off from his department in Nottingham to work with the secretariat to produce the documentation to win the political argument. An important document, *The work of the British Paediatric Association 1994*, was a 16-page booklet illustrating the range of activities of the BPA, which gave the reasons why college status was appropriate:

- The medical care of children is a discipline distinct from medical care of adults.
- The nation needs a body that speaks for the health needs of and health services for its children.
- The health service needs a body to promote the practice of paediatric medicine and to encourage doctors to train as paediatricians.

The contest to succeed David Hull as president involved five candidates, and it was the one most closely identified with the campaign for college status, Roy Meadow, who won. He had proposed (and lost) the motion that the BPA should become a college, at the AGM in Lancaster in 1973, and now, more than 20 years later, had the opportunity to make it happen.

But the opposition continued. The Privy Council had made clear that we had an uphill task and that we needed the support of other colleges and of influential people in the medical establishment. There were three outstanding difficulties that kept arising during the negotiations with the Privy Council and the Department of Health:

1. That the BPA did not (and perhaps could not) fulfil all the duties of a Medical Royal College. This was true, partly because BPA members usually were doing that work on behalf of one of the RCPs. Moreover, the BPA could not be responsible for medical examinations until it was a college and had the right to run such examinations. However, steps were taken, often to the annoyance of the London RCP, to ensure that the BPA controlled and ran as many of the tasks of a college as possible. A Continuing Medical Education (CME) programme was established by the Academic Board; the foundations of a Joint Paediatric Training Committee were established from the Specialist Advisory Committee in Paediatrics; regular separate meetings of Regional Advisers in Paediatrics were set up; District Paediatric Tutors were appointed; a full consultation and nomination process was established for the recommendation of Merit Awards; the Health Services, Manpower and Research Divisions were expanded. Thus, the BPA was able to say that it was fulfilling college tasks for paediatrics and child health as fully, and rather better than the three RCPs, and could do so more effectively because it represented the whole UK.
2. A second problem was that a substantial, and influential, minority of members did not wish the BPA to become an independent college. However, the size of that minority declined dramatically about the time of the public quarrels with the London RCP in early 1995, which are described later. When under attack, members unite and forget their differences.
3. The third obstacle was that other colleges and influential medical organisations did not appear to support our petition.

Ammunition was needed. Support was required from other medical organisations, and there had to be no opposition from the Department of Health or any part of government.

Rallying Support

A letter setting out our aims, together with *The work of the British Paediatric Association 1994*, and a summary of the case for a college, was sent to the presidents of all Medical Royal Colleges, and the major medical organisations, with a request for a letter of written support which could be forwarded to the Privy Council. Suitable letters of reply were few. Longstanding friends and supporters, such as the Royal College of General Practitioners (RCGP) and the Royal College of Obstetrics and Gynaecology (RCOG), sent cogent letters of support. Some other colleges with which paediatricians had thought they had good working relationships were not able to provide letters of support. Their president usually telephoned or wrote a personal letter to say how sorry they were that despite their personal sympathy for the cause, their council would not endorse a letter of support for a Paediatric College.

Successive BPA presidents had kept the presidents of the RCPs closely informed about what was happening. On taking office in 1994, the new president sought to gain the support of Professor Turnberg, president of the RCP London. Support was not forthcoming. However, the support of the two Scottish Colleges (RCP Edinburgh and RCPS Glasgow) was an important factor at a time when so many of the ancient colleges were very nervous of another new college diminishing their own prestige, power and income. The case was presented at the Conference (Academy) of Medical Royal Colleges – the meeting of all college presidents. Several seemed to fear that a Paediatric College would seek to attract members from them (e.g. paediatric surgeons, child psychiatrists, intensivists). The then chairman (Turnberg) was in a strong position and advised the meeting not to endorse the proposal. The president sent out a further series of letters, together with full documentation, to paediatric organisations abroad and to over a hundred professional organisations and charities concerned with children, seeking their written support, for delivery to the Privy Council. The response was overwhelming; it was clear that most of those organisations had the greatest respect for the BPA, valued its work and supported change that would enhance that work. Paediatric organisations in Europe and beyond pointed out how the UK was out of line with most of the world in failing to recognise paediatrics as a major specialty.

In the continuing discussions with the Privy Council, it became clear that the lack of support from the London RCP was a major obstacle. Other specialties had achieved college status after an interim period as a faculty of a parent college and usually with the support of that college. The Privy Council seemed to view the BPA as a rebel group within the RCP. Letters of support for our petition were numerous, but the Privy Council seemed to pay great attention to the letters of opposition, whether they be from a few former officers of the BPA or from the ancient and influential colleges. Even the Department of Health seemed nervous of the ancient colleges.

Opposition Unites Members of the BPA

Paradoxically, the opposition of the RCP became helpful. In the winter of 1994, the RCP president formally responded to the Privy Council opposing the petition. This letter infuriated many paediatricians who, themselves, were fellows of the RCP, because it seemed that the president was expressing the RCP view, without consulting its governing body comitia or its elected council (where the issue had not been discussed).

More than 1,400 people attended the BPA meeting in York in 1995. There was a very large attendance for the AGM and much anger and concern expressed then, and subsequently, regarding the RCP's response to our petition. Some of the more vociferous members suggested that paediatricians should resign from the RCP or take other retaliatory action. The opposition of the RCP, and the way in which it had been presented to the Privy Council, had united BPA members in support of the proposed college to an extent that seemed unlikely 6 months earlier. Members made it plain that they wished Council and its President to press our case to become a college urgently. By now the BPA had 3,300 members, a third of whom were consultants; the demand for college status was strong.

The strength of feeling within the BPA became known to the RCP where, in June 1995, its council discussed, for the first time since the submission to the Privy Council, the issue of an independent College of Paediatrics. Each of the five paediatric representatives, including the paediatric vice president and censor, explained why they now believed it is necessary for them to be a separate College of Paediatrics (two of them explaining that in the past they had not held that view). The paediatricians emphasised that they intended to work closely with physicians and that the formation of a college should lead to improvement in relationships, rather than the reverse. As was usual at RCP Council, no vote was taken. After the council meeting, the president of the London College wrote suggesting a new working party between the BPA and the college to explore 'new initiatives, such as formation of a Faculty'. BPA Council, meeting a few weeks later, had no enthusiasm for yet another working group. It was fully aware of the considerable efforts that had been made in the past to create a faculty and its rejection by the BPA membership. Paediatrics was a mainstream specialty, both in undergraduate and in postgraduate training, and should be represented by a college.

The regional advisers who acted for both the BPA and the Colleges of Physicians, and many of whom had great loyalty to the ancient colleges, nevertheless recognised the changes that had taken place in the structure of paediatric training and the need for paediatrics to be represented, as of right, on the Academy of Colleges. They expressed their unanimous support for a formal letter from them to the Privy Council in support of the petition. It was a persuasive letter, signed by many senior paediatricians who had the closest links with the three RCPs, many of whom were, or had been, office holders or council members of the three RCPs.

The Department of Health had a key role in advising the Privy Council. Several private meetings were held with the Chief Medical Officer (CMO), Dr Kenneth Calman, and others in the department. The CMO was identified with the creation of shorter structured medical training (Calman Training) and involved in the complicated legislation to oversee it and the creation of the Specialist Training Authority (STA). It was unthinkable that paediatrics would not be represented on the STA, and yet the rules proposed that only colleges should be represented, not associations of specialists. Our response was that the BPA should become a college and thereby become a full member of both the Academy of Colleges and the Specialist Training Authority. The CMO was a sympathetic listener ('in listening mode' as he called it), but made no promises. The DoH informed me that its papers would be placed before the relevant ministers at the end of the summer and that the Privy Council would then be advised.

The impression was that not only Dr Calman but also other members of the Department of Health had great respect for the work of the BPA and had no doubt that in relation to matters of child health, the BPA was the appropriate organisation with which to deal, thus acknowledging that in many ways the BPA already fulfilled the role of a medical Royal College. On the other hand, the department was involved in difficult negotiations within the European Union in relation to the creation of the Specialist Training Authority. In this work, they were assisted, and to some extent led, by Sir Leslie Turnberg, the current chairman of college presidents. There was an understandable reluctance to overrule him on the Paediatric College when he was such a far sighted, wise and effective leader on the European issue (Fig. 1.1).

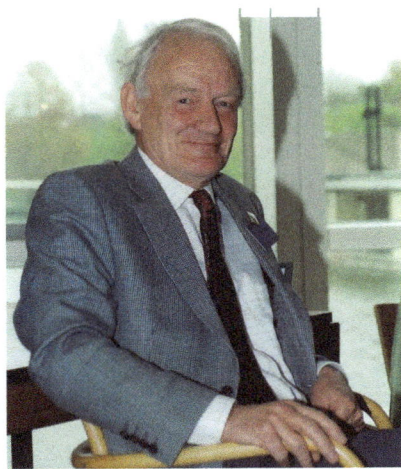

Professor Sir David Hull

Successful Conclusion

Lobbying at Westminster, at medical meetings, in journals and with professional colleagues at home and abroad continued. There was genuine uncertainty about the outcome and considerable foreboding. Then, in January 1996, a letter was received from the clerk to the Privy Council:

> The Privy Council, having considered the petition, are minded, without prejudice to recommend to Her Majesty that a charter be granted.

The news arrived during a meeting of the academic board. Champagne replaced orange juice at lunchtime. There followed a busy period in which the charter and bye-laws for our new college were refined and approved by the council.

Perhaps the last major argument concerned the title. Those of us who favoured a new college had, from the beginning, believed that it should be more than a union or society of paediatricians but also an organisation that promoted the health needs of children. Traditionalists wanted a 'College of Paediatricians' which would have been in line with every other medical Royal College, making clear that it was a college of specialists. However, the council agreed that we would seek a 'College of *Paediatrics and Child Health*' and that we would seek the approval of that title from our members at the AGM. As expected the debate was vigorous, but there was an over-whelming vote in favour of the longer, and more holistic, title. The battle was not quite over. Several other colleges, presumably mindful of the potentially high profile of a College of Paediatrics and Child Health, objected to the title, but at the meeting of college presidents, it was easy to point out that it was the business of paediatricians, not other specialists, to decide what their college was called and that paediatricians would not suggest alterations to the title of colleges other than their own. The move for the Academy of Colleges to intervene with the Privy Council was resisted. The College of Paediatrics and Child Health received its charter on 23 August 1996.

The appellation 'royal' comes on the recommendation of a department within the home office and is separate from the granting of a royal charter. Our initial charter was for a College of Paediatrics and Child Health. Previously, we had submitted papers to the home office requesting that it would be appropriate for us to be a 'royal' college from the beginning, rather than to be on probation for several years before achieving the royal appellation, as has happened to other medical colleges. The argument was accepted, but administrative problems within the government caused a delay of 2 months, until 17 October 1996, before we were entitled to use the present full title. Almost as if to confirm that final maturity, Her Royal Highness the Princess Royal graciously agreed to become our first patron.

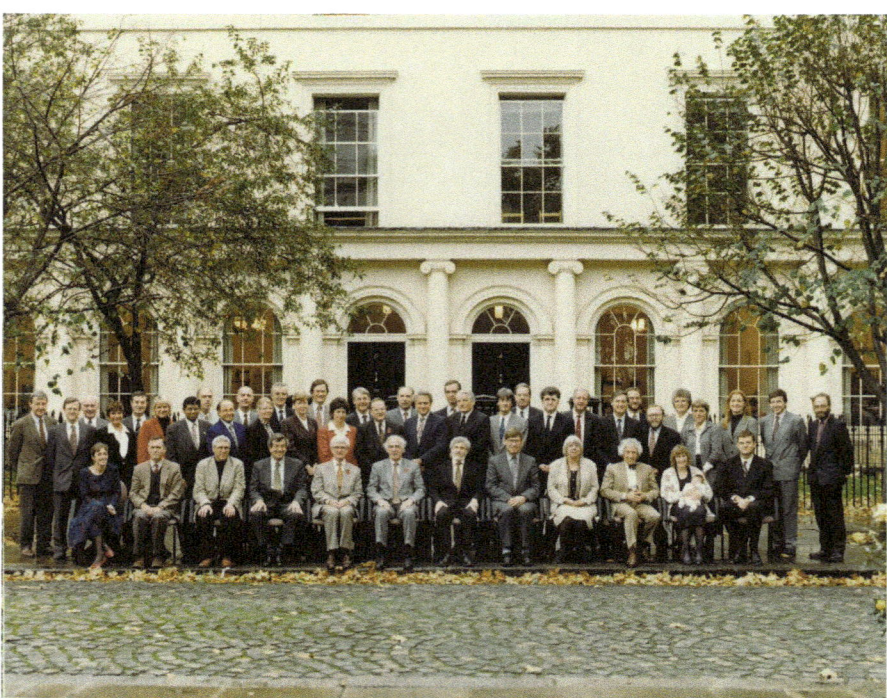

First meeting of RCPCH Council

Commentaries

2

Bertie Leigh, Dame Margaret Turner-Warwick,
Lord Turnberg, John Cash, Ian Lister Cheese,
Bernard Valman, Peter M. Dunn, and Timothy Chambers

As will be apparent, the road to becoming a separate college was long and rocky. Early paediatricians owed their main allegiance to the colleges which had looked after them during their training, and virtually all had passed the membership examination of one of these colleges and most were fellows. The Edinburgh College of Physicians for many years had a paediatric option for part of the clinical examination, but it was not until the early 1970s that the MRCP (UK) came into being with a common exam for all three colleges. There was a single UK-wide MCQ as part one with a set number of 'overlap' questions straddling the paediatric/adult interface. As will be seen in Chap. 9, this evolved into a completely separate paediatric examination. There was therefore a growing cohort of consultant paediatricians who did not have the same loyalty to a single ancient college and who saw themselves as an evolving specialty in their own right.

We have asked some of those who were intimately involved in the final process of separation to comment on what went on.

B. Leigh (✉) • L. Turnberg • B. Valman
London, UK

Dame M. Turner-Warwick
Devon, UK

J. Cash
Edinburgh, UK

I. Lister Cheese
Abingdon, UK

P. M. Dunn • T. Chambers
Bristol, UK

© Springer International Publishing Switzerland 2017
A. Craft, K. Dodd (eds.), *From an Association to a Royal College*,
DOI 10.1007/978-3-319-43582-4_2

The Legal View, Bertie Leigh

Bertie Leigh

Bertie Leigh was the solicitor for the BPA and the RCPCH. He is a senior partner at Hempsons Solicitors.

Around 1980, Charles Butcher, who was preparing for his retirement, asked me to take over advising the BPA. Hempsons had looked after them for donkey's years, but it was not seen as a very adventurous client. A bit of charity advice: they might want to amend their articles, but nothing is very interesting. Charles and I were already doing the most interesting and difficult paediatric work in our advice to the Medical Defence Union whose paediatricians brought us the most extraordinary profound issues which had not yet become the focus of public attention. We also advised on child protection to the National Society for the Prevention of Cruelty to Children. That was how I first became involved in the fascinating legal and ethical issues that were to occupy the rest of my career.

It was also through my work for the MDU that I came to know David Hull. He took over from Robert Illingworth as the paediatric member of the MDU Council, and we became firm friends, partly because I came to regard him as an almost infallible guide and partly because of his charmingly laconic way of describing people and problems. He talked to me about the problem of the BPA. It was an odd sort of arrangement, with a professional association for paediatrics wholly outside the Royal College of Physicians, which was supposed to represent, examine and govern them. This did not make it unusual in British medicine. The anaesthetists had had their own association administering a diploma since 1929, 20 years before the surgeons created a faculty for them so as to enable the new NHS to offer them posts of consultant status. So they had two examining bodies, one of which acted as a trade union and both of which provided some teaching. There were various other professional associations – such as orthopaedics and cardiology who represented groups of college members in external organisations, whose existence illustrated a need that at some time had been perceived as unmet by the broader college, but none of which felt it necessary to set up their own rival colleges. Those that had were obstetrics and gynaecology, radiology, pathology and ophthalmology, most of which had been represented by my firm.

Paediatrics was different as I learned from David for all sorts of reasons. First it cut across all the other colleges and specialties. Why should paediatric physicians be separate from adult physicians if not paediatric surgeons? If you split the cardiologists, nephrologists and gastroenterologists – what June Lloyd called collectively the 'offal specialties' – how would each paediatric group achieve a critical mass? Would they have to carry on being members of two colleges if they were going to treat some adults, as most still did?

The BPA was itself a self-selecting group of doctors who worked with children. Many members did not have the MRCP and so would not be qualified to be appointed as consultants. Many of them were employed working in schools or by local authorities looking after healthy children. There was not much linking those employed to do school inspections of children with the state-of-the-art specialists who were being appointed to run the first generation of neonatology units up and down the country. The name of the college itself represents the dichotomy between looking after children when they fell ill and needed hospitalisation and enabling children to grow up healthy. Would a Royal College admit these less academic doctors to membership on the same terms, and if it did, would it not devalue the coinage? How would you avoid paediatrics being seen as a soft option? Was there not an honourable role for the BPA that could not easily be done by a Royal College?

There was also the argument about Balkanisation. Splitting up the established Royal Colleges would replace one voice with a cacophony. The government would not like it because they would have to consult more than one body. Indeed, when they do not want to hear what the profession has to say or when the profession should be speaking with a united voice – as when it should have told the government that the Lansley reforms were misconceived – it is easy for them to play off one group against another. The great power of the RCP, with its wealth, tradition and dignity, carried a degree of clout that the BPA would not be able to match for a generation.

David Hull was sensitive to all of these arguments and was by no means single-minded in his determination to see a new college. Looking back I think that the established order was on the back foot from the early 1970s when the MRCP for paediatricians became a distinct examination. Until then the paediatricians all had to train and qualify in adult medicine. Once the training and examinations separated, the RCP was in effect supervising two professions, and both had to believe in the benefit of the shared college. I think the Court report in 1976 represented more of a turning point than most people realised at the time. Then the NHS was generally winning – by which I mean that things were getting better and there was a confidence that they were going to get better every year. There were new chairs of paediatrics springing up. The gap between what is and what should be, the lodestone of success for any health service, seemed to be getting narrower, training was improving, and the senior registrars completing their training seemed then to be more skilled and wiser than their predecessors had been at the same stage.

Professor Court's report provoked a realisation that things were not changing nearly fast enough in paediatrics. And if this meant that children were being let down, many paediatricians saw themselves as having an obligation to change things. They were shocked to discover that these 24 % of the population were getting only 3 % of NHS resources. The amount that should have been diverted to children depended on how ill they were and how expensive the therapies available were, and the Court report also showed more was needed. Many paediatricians believed things had to change and that children's medicine needed a stronger voice.

There was also a sense that the establishment was London-centric. Court continued the powerful tradition founded by James Spence in Newcastle, and it is not by chance that Spence gave his name to the medal that is the highest honour the college can bestow. A number of provincial young Turks who were leading change became active proponents: David Hull as the foundation professor in Nottingham found allies in Peter Dunn and David Baum in Bristol, Roy Meadow in Leeds, Richard Cooke in Liverpool, David Hall in Sheffield and Keith Dodd in Derby who felt increasingly disappointed by the London College that represented them. The shortcomings of the set-up were less clear in London, which then had 13 teaching hospitals as well as Great Ormond Street, a children's hospital that was already adept at punching above its weight.

The stigmata of these tensions are still there. When I was instructed to draft the charter and the bye-laws, the founders of the college were determined that the sovereign power should be held by a broadly based nationally representative council. Over the last 20 years, the direction of travel has been in the direction of much smaller groups of people exercising the power of the trustees of a charity, with larger groups being involved to decide ethical and professional issues that have little to do with the management of the organisation.

There was also a generational issue. A lot of the young Turks felt that the RCPL was led by older doctors who did not share their concerns about a wide range of issues. Hence I was also told to ensure that no office holder could be someone who had retired from current practice. I pointed out that recently retired people could have a lot to offer in the way of experience and time that the electorate might value, and it did not seem to be sensible to tie oneself to a rule that would have denied the British people the leadership of Churchill during the war, but such advice fell upon the stony stuff. Very often young organisations bear the scars of their early struggles in rules that sometimes appear difficult to understand if you do not study the history.

However, none of that was very clear when David and I started talking, or even when I received a letter from Jean Gaffin, the executive secretary of the BPA dated 3 March 1987 sending me a paper on the future of the Association. The next stage was the AGM decision to poll its members, and on 30 September 1987, we got the result of the referendum: this showed a narrow majority for independence over a faculty within the RCP, 506 to 498. More importantly, only 71 voted for the status quo. Things were clearly on the move, and on 23 October, the council voted to set up a working group to explore both options.

I was not involved in the working group until a year later when David brought June Lloyd and Paul Dunn to see me. In 1988 the AGM voted for a college that would be 'interdependent' with the three RCPs. I never really understood what that meant, but it was clear that things had moved on in the last year. When I told my seniors, who had guided the radiologists and the pathologists, what we were planning to do, they gave me very clear advice. 'Tell them it will take 10 years and they must be prepared to drink tea until it is coming out of their ears'. The second bit of advice went down better than the first.

My visitors wanted to know what it meant to be a Royal College. I had to explain that they were proposing a whole series of different changes. First you had to start a new body called a college. This would be a new incorporated organisation ruled by its articles and bye-laws and a registered charity. The BPA was an unincorporated association. Then you had to get a royal charter. Then you had to get permission to call yourself royal. And there had to be sizeable intervals between each of those events. However, to make it more confusing, things did not have to be done in that order, and most of the rules and advice owed more to lore and opinion than any identifiable law.

A royal charter is in effect an act of the crown, albeit in the Privy Council rather than parliament. It is traditionally 'bestowed as an acknowledgement of achievement rather than in hope', words that were to haunt us since they are not at first blush consistent with an application from a body that does not yet exist. It was reasonable to insist that you had to show that you were going to be financially viable as well as a responsible feature of society. After it would not do for bodies with royal charters to be wound up insolvent all following after a few years, but the BPA had stable finances. The problem was to prove that the paediatric college would work professionally and that the state should intervene in a dispute between doctors.

This led to a discussion about whether the BPA could, like Rhodesia, announce a unilateral declaration of independence ('UDI') and simply call itself the College of Paediatrics. We could incorporate, and after a few years of achievement, we could apply for a royal charter. In theory there was nothing to stop this. The GPs had set up a company limited by guarantee in 1952, been given permission to call themselves a Royal College in 1967 and been given a royal charter in 1972. However, they had also made sure that they had neutralised the opposition first.[1]

UDI would not work for the paediatricians. How would we persuade the membership to transfer if we did not have the backing of the crown? The RCP would still own the examination with all the standard questions the paediatricians had prepared over years, and the new college might not be consulted by anybody. We would put everyone's back up, and if it did not work, it would harm the cause of children to speak with two voices. Better to assemble those arguments against UDI and to use them to huff the opposition off the pitch when they insisted the new college was unnecessary.

So we decided that we wanted a new college and that we wanted a royal charter at the same time. The argument about the charter would force the rearguard to engage and be defeated. We could use the fact that the BPA had been stable for 60 years to reassure the crown that the association was viable.

---

[1] See A History of the Royal College of General Practitioners, Ed Fry, Hunt and Pinsent; Pub MTP Press 1983.

But that would only get us a College of Paediatrics. To be able to use the royal prefix had nothing to do with getting a royal charter. Indeed it was donated by a different government department. To get it, you simply wrote a letter, to the Home Office for some reason, and they would ask the Queen, and if she was 'pleased to grant permission', that would be the end of the matter. Except convention suggested, they would probably say no at first. Another case of Bestowed in Acknowledgement of Achievement rather than in hope, like the charter. The Royal College of Surgeons had waited a century. The obstetricians and gynaecologists got their royal charter in 1929 and became a Royal College in 1947,[2] but they were helped by having the then Queen as an active patron. The GPs had waited 15 years, even though they got it before their charter.

However, there was a useful precedent in the anaesthetists who had got it all at once. They had been able to say that they had existed as a faculty of the RCS for 40 years, and since it was a division of a Royal College, it would be wrong to deny them. Nevertheless, I thought that they represented a weakness that we could exploit. How could you turn down the profession who cared for a third of the nation? However, all that lay far in the future.

I got in touch with a friend at the Privy Council who I had dealt with on other things, and he was very welcoming. He told me that it was the kind of case that would get nowhere unless we got the support of the new Department of Health (DH) and the ministers. It was harder than it would have been 20 years earlier when people were more liberal about letting people have their way. There was a tendency to frown on Balkanisation, because of the danger of specialities subdividing ad infinitum. The likely attitude of the RCP would be important, but their opposition not necessarily fatal – it would depend on our arguments. The Privy Council operated through committees: this one would be chaired by the Lord President who would act as referee, but the decisive voice would be Kenneth Clarke, the Secretary of State at the DH. He offered to take soundings if I was instructed to write a letter.

That did not happen. June Lloyd wanted to get the council of the BPA to discuss it first. The Working Party had also produced a first draft charter, and they wanted me to advise on the wording of it. I had to advise that the precise words of the charter were a technical matter and entirely secondary to the issues of principle. However, they thought it would focus their debates and so I had to advise on issues like whether the new body would need a statutory express power to hire and fire staff or defend legal proceedings.

In 1990 there was a proposal for closer union of the BPA with the college, I think in effect the BPA would be folded into the RCP and that was defeated by a massive majority.

Things warmed up again when Sir David Hull became president in 1991. We had a series of meetings at which we hammered out our arguments, and it was clear that

---

[2] See Twenty five Years, Shaw, RCOG.

the independent college option was now in the driving seat. The 1992 AGM resolved to organise a referendum, and this time 61.8 % voted for an independent college. In June the council instructed the officers unanimously to seek a charter.

So I arranged to bring my clients to Downing Street, and the best china was out for our first polite cup of tea on 29 September 1992.

The PC was both informal and reserved. They were always helpful and very easy to deal with but gave less away about who they were talking to behind the scenes. They gently talked through the problems and obstacles. They made it clear that they talked to 'advisors' – which we knew meant anyone in government they thought would be interested. In practice it meant the Department of Health and to a much lesser extent Department of Education. The Department of Health would ask others, and this would mainly mean the existing colleges, mainly the RCP.

The main argument we had to confront was that the BPA was so good and doing so well that we did not need collegiate status. It might be incongruous that the government would sometimes consult the 'Royal Colleges and the BPA', but that showed how we were already respected. And the RCP insisted that when they were consulted about paediatric issues, they always put it across to the BPA or the Committee of Paediatrics. So there was really no need to change. If we did it, there would be massive additional expense to enable the profession to speak with more than one voice.

Another problem was that we were not united. They knew that there had been a lively debate at the AGM at York when it had been debated. My clients insisted that it was a handful of conservatives. One of them, Tim Chambers, had written a strong leader in the *Lancet*.

We were gently told that there were serious obstacles ahead of us. Nevertheless it was clear that attitudes had hardened at the BPA. Over the next few weeks, we prepared a memorandum – it was drafted by David Hull to enable the Privy Council to take soundings. I advised on a couple of points, but it was very much his document, and he did the work on it. On 2 December, I submitted it to the Privy Council.

Reactions from other colleges were mixed. Stanley Simmons, President of the RCOG and chairman of the Conference of Royal Colleges, thought it was 'stone cold' and did not see how anyone could oppose it. The RCS of Edinburgh was sympathetic but on the whole feared it would create an awkward precedent. Crucially, the RCP was hostile. Their clearest expression I ever saw was a letter from the president, Professor Leslie Turnberg, replying on 18 March 1993 to Professor John Forfar. It was friendly and conciliatory, but he was clearly digging in his heels. There were extensive negotiations behind the scenes before the Privy Council organised a second set piece meeting with a representative of the DH who was doing the consulting for them. That meeting on 7 October 1993 reported that the consultations had been inconclusive. They had done their best but no clear consensus had emerged. It was resolved that we should submit our draft petition and draft charter to smoke out the opposition.

This meeting was the first time Roy Meadow was involved as the new president elect, and I was impressed by the clarity of his vision: if Sir David had always seen both sides of the question and had been chosen as leader when the BPA was less certain itself, Sir Roy, as he was to become, had been a committed advocate and was chosen at a time when his colleagues had come to share his view. This was important because it indicated that those paediatric voices in favour of the status quo were a long way from the mainstream.

The rest of that year was spent exchanging drafts of the formal petition for a charter and the draft charter and bye-laws. These were submitted to the Privy Council on 14 February 1994. The AGM considered them in April, and they were approved by 247 votes to 16 against. So I was pretty shattered when the Privy Council wrote to me on 12 May that the:

> draft documents had now been considered on an informal basis by the Privy Council's advisers. Following these consultations, I must advise you that the indications are that a formal Petition from the British Paediatric Association is unlikely to be favourably received in the short term.
>
> I realise this news will be a disappointment to your clients. If they decide nevertheless, to proceed with formal submission, we shall of course arrange for any Petition to be considered. This process as you know will involve publication of a notice for representations

Informally I was told the problems were the position of the RCP, doubts from the Chief Medical Officer about whether a separate college was preferable to a faculty, an overestimate of the strength of the dissidents and doubt about whether it was appropriate to remove the examination. Although the gambit of submission in draft had enabled them to avoid turning us down flat – which would have made it difficult for the council to consult on a substantive submission within the next few years – it was as discouraging as it could possibly be.

Usually when you lose a case, the lawyer expects the clients to be looking at best rueful, but not my friends. They pointed out that I had warned them, it would take years, and they were ready and willing for the next bout of tea-drinking. Never mind the vivid warning, we were going back straightaway. They wanted to understand why we had not submitted formally, and I had to remind them that it was a gambit we had agreed on to enable us to reapply if they turned us down. As a result, we held a council of war on 16 June 1994: Sir Roy, Dame June Lloyd, Christopher Nourse and Paul Dunn came to my office to give final approval to the documents that were sent that day.

On 24 October 1994, the Privy Council sent me back the comments from the dissidents, and they seemed a bit dull and predictable. The PRCP pointed out there were numerous overlaps with adult medicine, that the RCP included paediatricians and that things worked well as they were. The PRCS, Sir Norman Browse, supported him in opposing Balkanisation, saying we were a 'subset' of the RCP. The only new voice to me was Professor Cyril Chantler, the Principal of Guys and St Thomas's who said that members of the BPA came from different professional backgrounds and that fragmentation would not help. Drs Tim

Chambers and James Appleyard repeated the views that they had frequently articulated before. Dr J. M. H. Buckler, the Regional Dean in Leeds, agreed with Tim Chambers.

None of this was new or impressive, and the comparison with the vast quantity of material we had assembled gave me confidence. I fear that I completely failed to recognise that the PRCP had made a significant mistake: he had answered the proposal formally without taking the issue to Comitia. My clients took the view that this fatally undermined the RCP's position that when they were asked to comment on questions involving paediatrics, they answered after talking to paediatricians. They said it did not matter that the government put questions about children to the RCP, because they had a paediatric vice president who chaired a paediatric board, and that one of their four censors was a paediatrician. He said they had paediatric advisors in every region of the country and made the whole arrangement sound perfectly reasonable and based firmly on paediatricians.

If I failed to spot the dissonance, Professor Meadow was onto it like a terrier. Within the profession and the department, this was a major focus of the debate. Most of these discussions did not involve lawyers on the scene, but I did have numerous discussions with Sir Roy, whom I came to admire enormously. He had a clear vision of what would be best for children and a determination to go for it: I was very happy to be used as a sounding board with whom he could rehearse arguments, but this was his battle. With the Privy Council, I was involved in a few further tea meetings, but it became clear that the temperature was warming up. The meetings tended to be pressing us for questions about why we had chosen to do things as we had. There were more tactful suggestions on how we might improve the drafting. Eventually it became clear that we had won: as Sir Roy was told by one civil servant in mid-1995, 'now you are unstoppable'.

Thus, by the time we got the answer in January 1996, it was a bit of an anticlimax. The battle had been won over the previous months. Immediately I had to start on the next stage working formally with the Privy Council on the final versions of the charter and bye-laws. That took until June. At the same time, we had to confirm the approval of the Charity Commissioners: we had shown them things in draft, but any amendment could raise some issue obscure to the rest of us. We were after all transferring substantial assets and property away from a national charity. There were also problems to sort out transferring staff, leases, and contracts relating to equipment, like photocopiers. There was a trading company and occupational pension schemes (thankfully these were not yet recognised as the show-stopping liability they later became). We had to make sure we would not pay Stamp Duty.

However, there remained the royal prefix. I was determined that it should be royal from the start, if there were to be more talk of 'bestowed in acknowledgement of achievement', and I thought it would be delayed 10 years. This was a much less formal matter, simply writing a letter saying why it should be so. The trouble was there would be no dialogue – either the letter pleased, and you got it or it did not.

415 50541 002 7   26 February 1996

R.M. Morris Esq
The Criminal Justice Constitution Department
The Home Office
50 Queen Anne Gate
London SW1

Dear Sir

I have the honour of acting for the British Paediatric Association which has petitioned Her Majesty for the grant of a Royal Charter incorporating a College of Paediatrics and Child Health. The Privy Council have indicated that they are minded, albeit without prejudice to recommend to Her Majesty the Queen that a Royal Charter be granted.

The purpose of this letter is to ask if the College may be granted permission to call itself the Royal College at the same time as it is instituted, which we hope will be in July. We appreciate that until the College of Anaesthetists was accorded this signal distinction it had never happened before, but my clients feel strongly that it would be appropriate in their case as well.

I **enclose** a copy of our Petition so that you can see the general nature of the Association and the case which it makes. In the rest of this letter I will merely identify some of the points which ought to be made in support of this application and confront one or two of the objections which I anticipate may be raised.

1.   The Importance of Paediatrics

It is trite to say that paediatricians care for the health of a quarter of the nation. The range of skills which modern paediatricians have to bring to their work is probably wider and more taxing than in any other specialty. Paediatricians work in all spheres of medicine from preventive and community child health to highly specialised hospital practice. Whereas adult medicine is divided between many specialties, the District General Hospital paediatrician in many cases has to be a specialist in everything from neurology to nephrology. If the paediatrician gets it wrong the consequences may be much graver than in the case of an adult physician, because so much more of the patient's life lies ahead. The job is also harder because many of the patients are incapable of describing their symptoms and their diseases are frequently distorted through the prism of parental concern. In short, there are good arguments for saying that paediatrics can be the most taxing and the most important of the medical specialties.

2. The Importance of Child Health

As the title of the College will make clear, the paediatrician also has a responsibility to the healthy child. Society expects the paediatrician to give advice in many areas of modern life in the hope that our children will be safeguarded from accident and disease. It is vital that the advice is given with an authority which is evident to the uninformed. Those who know nothing of these matters may well make the mistake of supposing that a College which lacks Royal patronage, that soubriquet of authority in our society, is a self-appointed collection of doctors whose advice may be disregarded with impunity. The health of children, one of the most precious of society's aims, is an object so high that inadequacies in the case my clients make may properly be overlooked.

3. The Importance of the Title

It is obvious that it is a great honour for a College to be allowed to call itself a Royal College and the paediatricians are mindful of the exceptional dignity that would be bestowed upon their nascent College if this were to be awarded at this stage. But the matter goes beyond the dignity of the College and also touches upon the examination and the title of every young paediatrician. Members of the Association already control the examination which has to be passed by young paediatricians who wish to become Members of the Royal College of Physicians. As from 1997 the examination will be renamed to bear the title of the new College. Our clients strongly believe that it would be appropriate for the new qualification to include the word Royal to indicate the dignity of the specialty. We believe it would be incongruous and inappropriate for the paediatrician alone of the consultants in a new hospital to bear a title which in some way implies that they are members of an inferior College or that they have passed an inferior examination, when the examination is in truth of an equal standard to that which has been passed by their colleagues in adult medicine.

This is particularly true of candidates from overseas. People from all over the world travel to England to pass the examination in Paediatrics to become members of the Royal College of Physicians. Our clients believe that this is an important part of the work of a College, helping to raise standards of medicine in many countries. It is also part of a community of scholarship based upon a shared concern for children which is the warp and weft of our clients' world. At the moment there are young paediatricians in Africa and Asia who will travel to this country to become members of the Royal College of Physicians. Some of them have acquired Part I and will work over the following years to acquire Part II. For them to be told in the middle of their training that they will only acquiring membership of an "ordinary" College, even one incorporated by Royal Charter would be a sad disappointment. There must be some possibility that if there is no title of this importance, the tradition of training and examining candidates from Third World Countries will be undermined.

4. Is it unprecedented?

Our clients do appreciate that the case that they make is not the same as that made by the Anaesthetists, who could claim to be a College already, albeit within the Royal College of Surgeons. The title College we suggest was, in their case, somewhat artificial since they were not already independent. Our clients are in a strange position, having been an autonomous institution responsible for the management of a specialty since 1928, as the British Paediatric Association, and yet also having chosen to perform their examination functions through their membership of the Royal College of Physicians until this year. In reality we do not think it is the fact that the anaesthetists were already a College which was the justification for them being accorded this honour at their birth, but the importance and dignity of the specialty of Anaesthesia. We respectfully submit that for the reasons we have already mentioned in this letter this is matched in the case of our client.

It may be suggested that if this signal honour were to be done to the College of Paediatrics and Child Health, in some way the floodgates would be opened to many other applicants. In reality, there are no other prospective applicants: there are 12 other Medical Colleges, all of them "Royal". I do not think it has ever been suggested that one of them was unworthy of the title, and I cannot suppose that it will be in this case. The purpose of floodgates is so that they can be opened when it is preferable to the alternative and that means that an exception should be made when confronted with a wholly exceptional case. We respectfully suggest that such a case was presented by the College of Anaesthetists and is now presented by the College of Paediatrics and Child Health.

Yours faithfully
M A M S LEIGH
c.c. N.H. Nicholls, Clerk to the Privy Council

The formal royal charter was granted by the Queen in her Privy Council on 23 July 1996:

HER MAJESTY, having taken into consideration the said Report and the Draft Charter accompanying it, was pleased, by and with the advice of her Privy Council, to approve and to order, as it is hereby ordered, that the Right Honourable Michael Howard, one of Her

Majesty's Principal Secretaries of State, do cause a warrant to be prepared for Her Majesty's for passing under the Great Seal a Charter in conformity with the said Draft.

Still nothing came from the home office. Eventually I learned that it had been delayed in the DH where it got lost on someone's desk. As a result, we did not get it until 18 October 1996. I called Roy at once, and we had a little celebration at my club that evening when I formally handed over the letter. The next day, I started drafting all the amendments needed to accommodate the change of name.

Dame Margaret Turner-Warwick (PRCP London 1989–1992)

The discussions on whether paediatricians should set up their own college was part of a much wider set of arguments affecting medicine in the 1980s and 1990s, and this background is an important part of the history of the more specific paediatric question.

The Royal Colleges of the UK in the Late 1980s and Early 1990s

This was a critical time when the colleges had to decide whether they wished to largely remain remote from politics as many colleges had done for centuries or whether changes in management of the NHS (with Mrs Thatcher's white paper on the NHS) made it necessary for them to engage more directly with the government, politicians and their policies. They could not be represented by the BMA alone on these political issues because this body was primarily a trade union for doctors, whereas the colleges were primarily concerned with standard of care for patients and training standards for doctors. The RCP on my watch decided the college had to broaden its remit, and I know that many other colleges agreed.

In turn this meant that the colleges had to develop two distinct roles: one concerned their own speciality and constituents both internally and externally and the other required working jointly with other major disciplines in medicine to present a strong and coherent voice representing the medical profession as a whole – working with the other Royal Colleges and faculties as appropriate and also through the conference of all the Royal Medical Colleges (later the Academy).

At this time, medicine was changing with a rapidly increasing trend towards specialisation within all of the major disciplines of medicine, surgery, pathology, etc. Understandably each new specialty wanted its autonomy in managing its own affairs and was often more concerned with this than supporting the standing of the medical profession as a whole at a time when politicians were set on undermining the standing and authority of the profession. In consequence, there were strong pressures towards proliferation of separate bodies with a potentially dangerous fragmentation of the profession. This also inevitably caused tensions between the role of the Royal Colleges and their specialist committees and the National Specialist Societies and Associations.

The RCP developed policies to give greater recognition to these specialist groups and at the same time promoted cohesion between them to strengthen the college to protect the profession as a whole.

The three Royal Colleges of Physicians (RCP) (London, Edinburgh and Glasgow) attempted, not always entirely smoothly, to work more closely together. The single UK membership examination in the early 1980s was a notable example of successful working together.

On my watch at RCP, a quarterly meeting was established (i.e. the so-called Noah's Ark meeting because 'the animals came in two by two'!). The chairmen of each of the RCP specialist committees paired with the president of the relevant national specialist association. This brought the national associations together and into the college. They debated who should lead on various topics including such things as standards, audit, training, etc., and at the same time the college recognised the autonomy of the specialist associations on specialty-specific issues. Interestingly this dual arrangement seems to have proved very successful over the years, and this contrasts with the demise of the BPA, all of whose activities have been taken over by the RCPCH.

We also strengthened the number of largely independent faculties within the college. These had their own premises, presidents and councils and had responsibility for their own training programmes and examinations. Not least they had their own place as members of conference. The fact that they remained within the RCP greatly strengthened the latter's hand when it came to representing physicians across the profession when they had to deal with politicians, the BMA, the GMC or other bodies.

It also became increasingly evident that the historical way that the medical profession was divided up between the colleges was in some ways becoming an anachronism, because of the ways in which medicine had advanced. This led to a number of regroupings.

Joint committees were set up between colleges. For example, RCP and microbiology within RCPath was developed to cover infectious diseases and another between RCP and RCR to cover oncology. Currently the RCP and RCGP are working very closely to improve the links between primary and secondary care. Some of the national associations also contributed to such regrouping. Thoracic surgeons and physicians came together as members of the British Thoracic Society just as paediatric respiratory physicians do now. Thus, there were a number of different ways that enabled different groupings of doctors from different colleges to work together when a new structure was required.

In spite of their efforts to regionalise, some of the colleges (perhaps especially the RCP) were regarded by the country at large as too London based and too remote. This stimulated a feeling of disenfranchisement among some specialities and in turn contributed to pressures towards proliferation of autonomous colleges in a number of different specialties.

Although RCP Council at the time agreed to its formation, I personally felt that the formation of the College of Accident and Emergency Medicine was not the right way forward because it set a precedent for fragmentation with a separate college for each medical, surgical, etc., specialty. This fragmentation of the medical profession was dangerous at a critical time when it needed to unite and speak with a single voice. Such fragmentation also opened the door for others including politicians to divide and rule.

RCP and Paediatrics in the Early 1990s

All these wider issues were very relevant to the discussions regarding the autonomy of paediatrics, which had continued since the 1970s and continued for some 25 years. There were strong reasons for staying within the RCP and equally understandable ones for wishing to separate. Some paediatricians wanted their own college, while others as fellows of the RCP believed in the strength of physicians caring for children and adults remaining together. It was regrettable over much of this time that the differences between RCP and many paediatricians became acrimonious.

Medicine in different age groups has many things in common and also many distinctions:

(a) Patients under the age of 12 years need very different management from those in their twenties, but these too differ from those over 70 or 80 years.
(b) Many adult diseases start in childhood.
(c) Many childhood conditions continue into adult life.
(d) Genetic disorders are lifelong, but the age of clinical presentation is often very variable.

On the other hand, as paediatrics evolved, the requirement for medical experience in older age groups was considered to be less important, and specialisation was introduced at a progressively earlier stage. Thus, as younger paediatric consultants increased, so their dissociation from adult medicine increased.

There are of course many other arguments in favour of separation, but these are outside my remit.

Because of all these and at the same time recognising the special position of paediatrics, the RCP made a number of suggestions in attempts to satisfy the need for paediatric autonomy without fragmentation of medicine by age groups:

(a) To form a *Faculty of Paediatrics* with its own president and council responsible for standards, examinations specialist committees, etc., the BPA could be restructured into a faculty with very little change. The concept of largely autonomous faculties within colleges had worked very successfully for public health (community medicine) and for occupational health.
(b) On my watch, the whole structure of the college was revised into four boards, i.e. for finance, education and exams, clinical medicine and paediatrics. The chairman of the paediatric board (who was also president of the BPA) was made a vice president of RCP alongside the vice president senior censor who became chairman of the education and examinations board. This substantially raised the status of paediatrics within the college.

Both of these proposals would have provided autonomy for paediatricians when they wished or needed to work independently, while allowing physicians for children and adults to work together as a single strong body when equally necessary. Sadly both proposals were rejected.

The Role of the Academy of the Royal Colleges and Its Predecessor the Conference of Medical Royal Colleges

This body could be very powerful in representing the medical profession as a whole, not as a trade union for doctors but representing the corporate view on standards of care for patients and standards of training for junior doctors.

Essentially it was for the presidents of the 13 or so Royal Colleges of the UK and their faculties to present a coherent voice of the medical profession to other public bodies.

For it to work successfully, members held the responsibility of presenting the collective opinions of the medical profession as a whole and thus worked together rather than the presidents being limited to the specific internal interests of their own particular councils.

Obviously this body could work more effectively if the numbers of representative bodies was limited and if the size of each was reasonably similar. Its work would become more difficult if the numbers proliferated too greatly and if they did not wish to consider matters beyond those of immediate relevance to their own college.

Its primary purpose was to present the views of the medical profession from the Royal Colleges and their faculties. My own opinion, perhaps borne out by events is that its influence was compromised by the later inclusion of representatives from other organisations, e.g. GMC, BMA, etc. Discussions on certain issues with other bodies were very important but have often confused debates which primarily concerned the Royal Colleges alone.

In my view, there is still major work for the academy to do in order for it to work optimally if the medical profession is to regain influence with government, the NHS and other major bodies. Without the unified voice of the Academy, the standing and influence of the profession will be greatly diminished and that will have grave consequences for patients and the medical profession alike.

Lord Turnberg (PRCP London 1992 to 1997)

It was the existing close relationships between physicians and paediatricians that prompted me to try to resist the split. Paediatricians had always been a strong force for good in the RCP, and developments in many of the specialties for which we were responsible often went hand in hand. With a paediatric vice president, a paediatric membership exam and large numbers of Fellows, paediatrics was more strongly represented in the RCP than any other discipline, with June Lloyd, David Hull and John Dodge as successive vice presidents and Robert Boyd as academic registrar. I could not see the loss of such valued colleagues with much equanimity.

But perhaps the most cogent reason for wanting to avoid a split was the problem of the increasing number of colleges vying for the ear of the government. Negotiations about such common matters as medical education, the health service, medical research and the increasingly intrusive messages coming from the EU meant that the colleges had to speak with one voice if they stood any chance of being heard. Further splintering did not seem to me to be a way in which the colleges would be strengthened even though paediatricians themselves might be given the freedom to manage their own affairs. The subsequent relative weakness of the Academy of Medical Royal Colleges (AoMRC) has indeed allowed the government either to ignore the colleges or play one off against the other.

In the end of course we bowed to pressure and since my motives had always been to work as closely as possible with our paediatric Fellows, I was very keen that good working relationships should be developed between our two Colleges. It would have been perverse to do otherwise, and it is why I was very supportive of the proposal that the Royal title be applied as soon as possible.

I was particularly gratified to be invited to give the after dinner speech at the first annual meeting in York and, as I said at the time, the fact that I was there was 'a marvellous demonstration of the human capacity for forgiveness'.

Since then your college has prospered and fulfilled its responsibilities with great distinction. It is a pleasure to acknowledge your achievements.

Professor John Cash, PRCP Edinburgh (1994 to 1997)

As president of the RCPE I was made aware of the 'big debate' by John Forfar, Professor of Child Life and Health in Edinburgh, who was then President of the BPA. He came in to brief me on the work of his committee and after a lengthy briefing, I came to the conclusion that he was deeply unhappy with the situation, especially around the role, and perceived power of the RCPL and its then president Les Turnberg.

I advised John that if the primary interest was the quality of the future practice of paediatrics in the UK and in effective training and training validation programmes, then he had made more than an adequate case for me to add my support for an independent College of Paediatrics and Child Health. I further advised him that I thought the current RCPE Council would support this development.

While welcome, this expression of support seemed to cause some discomfort which seemed to be related to the perceived power and influence of the RCPL and its President. He believed that this view was shared by many paediatricians as the President of the RCPL had a uniquely influential role in advising government on health policy development and in the selection of doctors for distinction awards and civil honours. He expressed the concerns voiced to him that standing out against the PRCPL could bring retribution.

I had worked very closely with the other two RCPs and had observed that the apparent omnipotence of the RCPL could be successfully challenged and frequently was. I was aware that when the two Scottish RCPs challenged the RCPL, it could cause both surprise and irritation.

Some weeks after my briefing by John Forfar, I spent time discussing the matter with Les Turnberg. I was surprised, and somewhat alarmed, at the emotionally charged reaction I received. He seemed particularly concerned with the emergence of societies representing the professional interests, including training, of emerging medical specialties. He felt clear that these developments would threaten the future viability of the ancient Royal Colleges. He reminded me of the way that Sir John Dacie had walked out of the RCPL, taking haematology to the RCPath. He viewed the demands of the paediatricians, if met, would open the flood gates for cardiology, respiratory medicine and gastroenterology, etc. I did not share these concerns, and, if he was so concerned, why had he not supported the RCPE proposals for the development of joint RCPUK specialty exit examinations? On being asked whether he thought there would ever be a paediatrician president of the RCPL, his answer was an unequivocal 'no'.

It was later in 1995 that Naren Patel (president of the RCOG) invited the presidents of the Scottish Royal Colleges to join him for an informal dinner and discussion at the RCOG. It was during this dinner that he revealed that the day before the meeting of all the college presidents at the Conference of Medical Royal Colleges, the presidents of the RCPL, RCSE, RCOG and RCPath would meet to discuss the forthcoming agenda and decide on positions to take. If problems were foreseen, then other college presidents were contacted with a view to achieving a satisfactory majority in any upcoming vote. The RCPL took the lead in convening this group of four presidents. There was never any doubt in my mind that the president of the RCPL had substantial influence on his other presidential colleagues, and I was not surprised that they did not promote the cause of the paediatricians.

Dr Ian Lister Cheese

Towards Establishment of the Royal College of Paediatrics and Child Health: A Recollection from the Department of Health

Dr Ian Lister Cheese was the Department of Health's internal paediatric adviser during the period when College status was being discussed. Here he gives some important insights into the DH role.

The case for establishing a College of Paediatricians had been set out in a memorandum from the BPA in 1992. This had been prepared during the previous year under the leadership of Professor (later Sir David) Hull, president of the Association (1991–1994). It brought up to date the medical professional and health services background to the thinking of paediatricians.

The essential reasons were that paediatrics was a distinct discipline, that paediatricians needed their own training programmes and standards in the practice of paediatrics and child health and that the BPA already had many of the responsibilities that in other medical disciplines fell to the colleges.

Formal involvement of the Department of Health in the journey to the grant of a royal charter establishing a college began in February 1994 when the Privy Council submitted a draft petition for comment.

The Department acknowledged that the BPA had made a strong case for seeking college status, but held that it was not an overwhelming case. It did not question the capability of the proposed new body to fulfil the duties and responsibilities required and expected of a college. Initial reluctance to support the petition was based chiefly on three factors: that it was unconvinced that the results of ballots conducted by the BPA were sufficient to demonstrate the support of most paediatricians; that the Royal College of Physicians, which represented a large number of paediatricians and paediatric interests, withheld its support; and that the BPA had given insufficient consideration to faculty status within the Royal College (or colleges) of Physicians.

At this time and subsequently the department expressed a broader concern that further differentiation (often called fragmentation) of the disciplines and specialties to form new collegiate bodies would not be in the best interests of the profession.

Meanwhile, putting aside this discouragement, in July 1994, the BPA submitted its petition to the Privy Council.

The perceived consequences of continued differentiation of the medical profession were that an increase in the number of colleges could lead to a weakening of the position of particular specialties and also make official consultations with the profession more complex. It was not at all clear how or why the position of particular specialties might be weakened, but the question arose at a time when EC Directives on training for specialist practice were being implemented following the recommendations of the Calman Report.

In due course, the proposal to establish a unitary competent authority for specialist medical training – on which the colleges would be represented and with which the department would increasingly deal – would reduce this risk. Indeed, the formation of a paediatric college would facilitate the implementation of the Calman Report in this specialty.

A shared view of all the health departments was that it would be preferable, as a first step towards independence for the BPA to form a faculty within the Royal College of Physicians of London but was not acceptable. It had been rejected by the BPA, partly on the grounds that many paediatricians were not members of the college. Moreover, it would not be acceptable to the Scottish colleges for all paediatricians to be members of a Faculty of the London College. The option of a joint faculty was considered but rejected by BPA members.

Within the department, a minority of officials were Fellows of the RCP or members of the BPA, or of both bodies, providing diverse sources of advice and participation in discussion. Although unsurprising, it should be recorded that discussion was restrained, uncoloured by the emotion and ferocious debate witnessed among those who would be most directly affected by the result.

A minor diversion was the question of choice of title – College of Paediatrics and Child Health. It was necessary to emphasise that the title had been chosen deliberately to reflect that the overriding aim was to serve children, not just the interests of its members, and that the petition concerned doctors in the field of paediatric medicine and child health and the objectives did not encroach on matters which were the responsibilities of other professions.

It might reasonably be thought that initially the Department, though properly concerned by the opposition of the RCP and some other medical Royal Colleges, and notwithstanding the results of the BPA ballots, feeling unsure about the balance of paediatric opinion, gave undue weight to the possible consequences of further differentiation of the collegiate bodies and too little to the strength of the case presented by the BPA.

During 1995 there were shifts in opinion. By August it had become evident that objections previously held against the establishment of a college had lessened. The petition had the support of the Royal College of Physicians and Surgeons of Glasgow and the Royal College of Physicians of Edinburgh. The President of the Royal College of Physicians of London, although at first unpersuaded of the case, no longer objected to the grant of a charter. Importantly, other senior physicians who had opposed separation from the RCP, while regretting the prospect of a separate collegiate body in paediatrics, no longer opposed it and would give all their support to a new college in its endeavour.

Although there remained a view within the department that a further referendum by the BPA was desirable as a means of affirming more convincingly the wishes of the current membership, events made this step unnecessary.

In November 1995, the department wrote to the Privy Council to say on behalf of UK Health Ministers that it supported the BPA's petition to establish a Royal College of Paediatrics and Child Health.

Dr Bernard Valman

Bernard Valman was a paediatrician at Northwick Park and heavily involved with both the paediatric activities of the RCPL and the new college. For many years, he was editor of the Archives of Disease in Childhood and was the new college's first honorary archivist.

A Long Gestation

In 1943 Donald Paterson proposed the founding of a College of Paediatrics, but a decision was postponed due to the war. When the NHS started in 1948, Paterson returned to Canada, and the topic was not revisited until the 1970s. Donald Court (President of BPA 1973–1976) told me that when he tried to engage government departments to implement his report on the future of the Child Heath Service (1976), he was told that they would only accept representations from the Royal College of

Physicians (RCP) which included the paediatricians. As Court had no official standing in the RCP, there were considerable delays in the implementation of his proposals. A major change was the appointment of community paediatricians, which was opposed by the Faculty of Public Health of the RCP. Court was adamant that a College of Paediatrics was essential to improve the medical care of children. His successors as presidents of the BPA and their councils agreed, although the majority of the members were hesitant for several years.

The RCP gradually gave concessions to the paediatricians with a paediatric written paper and later a paediatric clinical examination in the MRCP, a paediatric representative where there were two delegates to a committee, a paediatric censor and a paediatric vice president. A house in the precinct opposite the RCP was provided for the BPA at a peppercorn rent. There was a paediatric representative on every College Committee as well as a Paediatric Committee which was attended by the president and registrar of the college. I was secretary of this committee from 1981 until 1991 and in 1982 was appointed editor of Archives of Disease in Childhood, the journal owned jointly by the BPA and the BMA. This gave me two allegiances which were partly resolved by Peter Tizard, the president of the BPA. He had recently been chairman of the Paediatric Committee of the RCP, and he invited Tony Jackson, who was the current chairman of the Paediatric Committee of the RCP, for tea at his ancestral home at Ickenham Manor. An oral agreement was made called the Ickenham Concord that the Paediatric Committee would discuss only internal matters such as the DCH and all requests for advice from outside bodies would be forwarded to the BPA. This was intended to avoid conflicting advice being given on behalf of paediatricians, but excluded the Paediatric Committee from any discussion about a future Paediatric College or making any contribution to the development of care for children. I tried to remain impartial by acting as a reporter rather than expressing my personal opinion.

In 1985 Mrs Thatcher introduced 'general management' and her own medical advisors who were independent of the colleges. The abolition of Regional Paediatric Committees with their chairmen, who were advisors to the Regional Medical Officers on priorities, removed the possibility of district paediatricians influencing the development of local services. Paediatricians became despondent at their inability to improve care and were persuaded that only a college of paediatrics would recognise and fight for the service that children and their families needed and deserved. They knew that a paediatric college would reduce the membership income to the RCP by about 25 % and might precipitate the demand for new colleges from cardiologists and other specialists, but they pointed out that paediatrics was unique in being a whole body specialty.

To assess the implications of an interdependent college, in 1989 the Paediatric Committee became a conduit to yet another committee which had members from the three Royal Colleges of Physicians and the BPA. The term interdependent was never defined, but the members of the new committee had to report back to their respective colleges for proposals to be ratified before implementation. This slow and ineffective process was abandoned and the College of Paediatrics and Child Health was founded when the Privy Council rescinded its opposition.

Peter M. Dunn

Professor Peter Dunn was a paediatrician in Bristol with a major interest in neonatology. He was a powerful and vocal advocate for a separate college.

The news in 1996 that the Privy Council had granted Royal College status to paediatrics and child health ended a debate within our discipline that had lasted more than 20 years. It gave me the greatest pleasure. My reasons for preferring college status rather than becoming a faculty within the Royal College of Physicians (London) were given in a memorandum on the future of the BPA that I wrote in 1984. The following is an extract:

'The BPA started as a paediatric club 55 years ago and slowly developed into a forum for the exchange of paediatric ideas and scientific progress. Only in the last 15 years has it attempted to exert political influence on behalf of children. This was necessary because of the failure of the RCP to fulfil this function. As the Court Report (1976) pointed out, in 1972–73 only 9 % of total health expenditure in this country was spent on children's health services, although they constituted 24 % of the whole population and, at that, a section of the community with special needs. A decade later it has been stated that the financial balance is even more unfavourable to the child health services (9 % → 4 %).

Although the BPA has made great strides in the political arena, it lacks the prestige and automatic direct entré to Governmental debate which is automatically accorded to the Royal Colleges. This only necessary to observe the present influence of the RCOG in comparison to that of the BPA (which was actually founded a year earlier).

It has been argued that paediatrics would attain the required political influence by becoming a Faculty in the RCP. This might be possible if general medicine also became a similar Faculty within the College. But no one seriously believes that this would happen. Thus, Paediatrics would, by becoming a Faculty, be designating itself as a sub-specialty of adult medicine and, more important, would make it in the long run even more difficult to lift children from the second class health status that they have today.

There is a stronger argument against paediatrics attempting to exert its influence through the RCP, which is derived from the nature of childhood. Children are not little adults, but growing, developing persons in their own right. The acceptance of this fact by parents, professionals and politicians is essential if children are to be given the status in society which guarantees optimum care. The nature of that care is far wider than ensuring links with adult medicine important though that is. It involves a range of professionals committed to improving the quality of child health and well-being and the strengthening of family life which alone can sustain this.

Our professional links are naturally with the RCGP, the RCOG, the RC Psych., Teachers and Educational Medicine, Health Visiting, Children's Nursing and with Community Physicians when concerned with the planning of Child Health Services.

In addition our vision and service will involve the Third World, which needs evermore to value children and child health in its communities.

A strong body of paediatricians committed to child health, and with the respect and authority a College would have, is central to the cohesion and effectiveness which such a professional opportunity and responsibility requires'.

The debate on the future of the BPA was evenly matched. Views were strongly held and expressed by both sides. However, by 1990–1991, a steadily growing majority of paediatricians favoured the creation of a college. From that time onwards, paediatricians united in their efforts to persuade the Privy Council, the RCP and others that child care and health required and deserved college representation. Roy Meadow's 'Winning the battle for a College' provides an excellent account of these later years. However, no doubt for diplomatic reasons, his account barely touches on the internal debate of earlier years.

In 2000 I bound my collected papers and correspondence into two volumes with the title 'The struggle for a Royal College of Paediatrics and Child Health, 1973–2000' and presented them to the new college. Because much of the correspondence therein was of a confidential nature, I requested that the volumes be embargoed until 2020 while granting access when required to college historians. I believe these volumes will, in due course, provide an insight to the vigorous debate that took place during the 1980s. The volumes were dedicated to Donald Court, Dick Smithells, Roy Meadow and David Baum who, with others, did so much to achieve our Royal College. Already its achievements vindicate the importance they and many others attached to its creation.

Timothy Chambers

Timothy Chambers is a paediatrician in Bristol who held office both as secretary of the BPA and as a member of Council and a Censor of the Royal College of Physicians of London during this time. He wrote an anonymous editorial to the Lancet in 1988 strongly against the formation of a separate college and was also one of those who wrote an oppositional letter to The Privy Council referred to in the chapter by Sir Roy Meadow. He was asked to comment on the formation of the college, his role in it and whether it was worthwhile.

Not all paediatricians were in favour of a separate college.

Sir Roy Meadow has written an elegant and eloquent chapter about how the college came into being during the 1990s. His involvement goes back to the beginning of the 1970s, and its establishment is a tribute to the single-mindedness and tenacity of his personal crusade. It is the greater for having been achieved despite the indifference or hostility of the majority of British paediatricians, expressed as voting members of the BPA. In his chapter 'Winning the battle for a College'[1] commented on the 1992 referendum where there was a majority of those who voted in favour of becoming a college although this was not a majority of those eligible to vote.

An alternative gloss might be that whereas a substantial, influential and persuasive minority wanted a college independent of the RCP, the majority either did not, was passively acquiescent, indifferent or undecided. Nevertheless, with impressive hard work (notably from Sir David Hull) and interesting politics the mood of the membership was set aside and the resources of the BPA mobilised to engineer its transformation into a college.

I was asked in 2013 to answer the question 'Was the battle worth it and has the RCPCH been a better voice for children and paediatricians than the RCPs would have been?' It is too early for me to tell.

It does seem that the attitude of the Department of Health (DH) had considerable influence over the outcome. Meadow describes its apparent ambivalence between 1992 and early 1996.

The Royal College of Paediatrics and Child Health was formed, and its presidents became sovereigns of their small kingdom. In 1996 Dr Richard Smith, then editor of the British Medical Journal (BMJ), wrote an editorial in the context of a perceived lack of leadership of the profession, not least from 'a 'blitzkrieg from the right' at the end of the 1980s'. Within Smith's piece was this:

> Meanwhile, the colleges have gone on splitting, and new committees with unmemorable acronyms have appeared to represent academic medicine. Medicine has many leaders but little leadership. 'There is no kingdom,' says John Green, chief executive of the Royal Society of Medicine, 'too small for a doctor to be king of.' More potentates means less influence.

Was the battle worth it? History does not permit trials, randomised or controlled. We know it consists in events. Who could say what might have been achieved if the paediatric establishment had thrown its wholehearted weight behind the RCPs when they were beginning to accept that paediatrics was not a specialty of internal medicine? Was my 1988 Lancet editorial prescient or pusillanimous to foresee the balkanisation of the medical royal colleges?

Are the medical Royal Colleges now important sub specie aeternitatis? All I would say is that if in 2016 the neonatologists wanted to remove themselves from the RCPCH and form their own college, I doubt if it would register at the DH, with senior NHS management or politicians. The colleges' job is to provide training and revalidation homes – at some expense (and the RCPCH has one of the more costlier college subscriptions) – for the medical workforce of the UK whose control of standard setting in education and service is largely nationalised. The running in UK healthcare is now made by central and devolved governments, their departments and agencies, determining policy in all spheres of UK medicine and increasing the regulation of doctors. The route to this diminished influence is interesting. In 1987, during one of the periodic spats between the profession and the politicians, three London-based Royal College presidents had this published in the BMJ.

On 7 December the presidents of the Royal Colleges of Physicians, Surgeons, and Obstetricians and Gynaecologists issued the following joint statement.

Each day we learn of new problems in the NHS-beds are shut, operating rooms are notavailable, emergency wards are closed, essential services are shut down in order to make financial savings. In spite of the efforts of doctors, nurses, and other hospital staff patient care is deteriorating. Acute hospital services have almost reached breaking point. Morale is depressingly low.

It is not only patient care that is suffering. Financial stringencies have hit academic aspects of medicine in particular, because of the additional burden of reduced University Grants Committee funding. Yet the future of medicine depends on the quality of our clinical teachers and research workers.

Face saving initiatives such as the allocation of £30m for waiting lists are not the answer. An immediate overall review of acute hospital services is mandatory. Additional and alternative funding must be found. We call on the government to do something now to save our health service, once the envy of the world.

SIR RAYMOND HOFFENBERG
IAN P TODD
SIR GEORGE PINKER

On 7th December war was thus declared. The result was considerable medico political jousting and consultations with ministers. It culminated in a presidential deputation to the prime minister. What followed is recounted in the RCPL's Munk's Roll entry for Hoffenberg (a big man, courageous and unflinching in politics (within and without medicine) and professional and intellectual affairs): Munk's Roll is the collection of biographies of all Fellows of the RCPL over the last almost 500 years and for Hoffenberg states:

> He clashed with Mrs Thatcher (Baroness Thatcher, the then Prime Minister) on more than one occasion. She was, he said, the only person in his career to render him speechless when, with the presidents of the Royal Colleges of Surgery and Obstetrics and Gynaecology, he visited 10 Downing Street to discuss grave concerns about the state of the NHS. They were told that she would deal with them as she had with the miners and the miners' leader, Arthur Scargill.

20 years later, who can say that she has not succeeded? During that time, there has been a proliferation of medical representative bodies – academies, colleges and faculties, running counter to the opinion of a former professor of paediatrics at the University of Cambridge that 'it would be anyway a good thing were the expanding universe of medical colleges to begin to contract'. Perhaps this is an inevitable reflection of the complexity and technology of medicine, changes in its status and its relationship with the general healthcare management/leadership culture.

Or, like Great Britain, has UK (or perhaps, English) medicine 'lost an empire and has not yet found a role'? In 2008 the authors of a BMJ Personal View called for an Institute of Medicine: two years later a multiprofessional College of Medicine was launched at the House of Commons, followed by a symposium at the Cabinet War Rooms – an intriguing venue. The 2000s have seen UK medicine reviewing, and enquiring into, medical professionalism and leadership: not symptoms of an organisation at ease with itself. Meadow reproduces Cooke's tactless letter which includes the sentence 'When is it going to stop?', perhaps with professional realignments leading to multiprofessional standard-setting bodies, not always based on the medical collegiate/faculty caste system.

In my personal summary of the College's performance for children and paediatricians, there have been welcome successes including:

- The large increase in number of members
- Respect in the family of colleges
- Work the college has sponsored abroad – the success of its educational initiatives in Palestine, promoted by the late Professor David Baum, a staunch and magnanimous champion for a college
- Empowerment of young people
- Involvement in the Medicines for Children Network
- Further development of the British Paediatric Surveillance Unit
- Taking responsibility for examinations (but see below)
- Close alliance with the European Academy of Paediatrics

Nonetheless, important opportunities may have been missed internally:

- Taking a fresh look at the expensive and disruptive membership examination: Nordic countries train good paediatricians without exams.
- Ways of contributing abroad to local needs for education and assessment without colonising with the MRCPCH examination.
- Instead of decanting some services to areas of less employment, thereby helping to relieve UK child poverty, the college has invested in larger London property.
- One paediatric specialist society has moved its link with the college to an alliance with the academic society of its corresponding internal medicine specialty.
- Paediatric cardiologists have not moved from the RCPs.
- Outcomes of medical care of UK children (surely a college imperative?) are worse than in other European countries, with concern about mental health in particular.

Despite the lack of self-certainty in its strap line 'Leading the way in Children's Health', to claim that the RCPCH has provided 'a better voice for children' (however that is understood) might be regarded by future historians as a shade premature.

A better voice for paediatricians? They might deliver an earlier verdict. Whether it would be for consolidation, like our Sri Lankan colleagues, who followed us and split from the physicians' college, or reconfiguration (the Australasian colleges of paediatrics and physicians amalgamated in 1998) only events will tell. However, they – especially the young – might be more sensible and wonder what all the fuss was about and why we cared, medical turf wars being so retro. So why did we confront each other, cutting across long-held friendships and professional loyalties – at some personal cost (the Geneva Convention does not cover the medical political battlefield)? Both sides held strong views including the place of paediatrics and its status in UK medicine, implications for trainees, medical royal colleges and their place within UK society, the status of children and young people in society and how they would be best served by the colleges. These were honourable and profound differences of opinion, principles and values which those on either side felt should be defended to the extreme. Would I do it again? Yes.

Whatever its future, the college's basic function is to safeguard the public interest and its health. It does this by standard setting of paediatricians, both trainees and consultants, through education and validation and medical services for children. These are heavy responsibilities, and to discharge them without distraction, it requires people of no less adaptability, vision and drive than those who engaged in the battle over the college. Our specialty does not want for them: as we look forward 14 years to the centenary of the BPA/RCPCH, I wish them well.

Sir David and Sir Roy, *si monumentum requiritis, circumspicite. Vos saluto.* If you look for a monument, see what you have made happen. We salute you (paraphrasing the inscription on the tomb of Sir Christopher Wren in St Paul's Cathedral – *Si monumentum requires circumspicite*).

Further Reading

1. Meadow R. Winning the battle for a college. In: Valman B, editor. The Royal College of Paediatrics and Child health at the Millenium. London: RCPCH; 2000.
2. Smith R. Does Britain need an academy of medicine? Br Med J. 1996;312:1374.
3. Anonymous. A college of paediatricians? Lancet. 1988;1:1030–1.
4. Hoffenberg R, Todd IP, Pinker G. Crisis in the National Health Service. Br Med J. 1987;295:1505.
5. Warden J. A lesson in realpolitik. Br Med J. 1988;296:368.
6. Ledingham JGG. Munk's Roll, vol. XII. Royal College of Physicians of London. http://munk-sroll.rcplondon.ac.uk/Biography/Details/5775.
7. Davis J. Who needs a college for obstetrics and gynaecology? Lancet. 1987;ii:1465.
8. Acheson D. Speech at West Point (5 December 1962), in Vital Speeches 1 Jan 1963 p. 163.
9. Minhas R, Patel KCR, Wierzbicki AS. The UK needs an institute of medicine. Br Med J. 2008;337.doi:10.1136/bmj.a1623 (Published 9 September 2008).
10. Wolfe I, Thompson M, Gill P, Tamburlini G, Blair M, van den Bruel A, Ehrich J, Pettoello,Mantovani M, Janson S, Karanikolos M, Martin McKee M. Health services for children in Western Europe. Lancet, Published online March 27, 2013. http://dx.doi.org/10.1016/S01406736(12)62085-6.
11. The UK is failing our most vulnerable children. Growing up in the UK -Ensuring a healthy future for our children. BMA; 2013 http://web2.bma.org.uk/pressrel.nsf/wall/A155E91BC1BADA6380257B6D002EE86D?OpenDocument.
12. Chambers TL. Feral children. J R Soc Med. 2002;95(9):429–30.

Regalia and Ceremonies

3

Bernard Valman

Shortly after receiving the charter for the RCPCH, Keith Dodd, the Honorary Secretary, told me that the executive committee had requested that I should enquire about the production of a coat of arms. David Baum, the President-elect, and I, the Honorary Archivist, were to make the arrangements. I phoned the College of Arms for advice and was put through to the Richmond Herald, who was duty herald for the day. After asking a few questions, he said that, provided that we were prepared to pay £7,000, there should be no difficulty. I made an appointment to meet him with David Baum, at the College of Arms, near St Paul's Cathedral. The ground floor contains a court where cases of dispute on heraldic matters can be heard. We went up the creaking wooden staircase lined with framed sheets of parchment containing coats of arms belonging to dynasties long dead.

The Richmond Herald, who with his half-moon spectacles resembled a friendly family solicitor, suggested that we should decide on the concepts that should be incorporated, bearing in mind that the coat of arms should be distinctive and easily recognised. We included the aims of the College, the history of British paediatrics and child health and some double meanings. Through the College newsletter, we asked members for suggestions, most of which were incorporated in the final design, which was approved by the executive committee without change.

The coat of arms was painted on parchment in time for it to be used on the programme for the first AGM of the new College in April 1997. The members were delighted with the design, apart from some Lancastrians who objected to the rose, which was white. We had chosen a white rose because it represented the city of York,

B. Valman
London, UK

© Springer International Publishing Switzerland 2017
A. Craft, K. Dodd (eds.), *From an Association to a Royal College*,
DOI 10.1007/978-3-319-43582-4_3

where many annual meetings had been held, as well as the rose of England. After consultation with the Richmond Herald, one of the white roses was repainted red.

There were three symbols with double meanings. The position of the child at the top represents a concept that paediatricians wish to be as altruistic as parents aspiring that the child reaches a level of attainment higher than their own. The tree of life (oak) represents child development and health and also refers to the first president of the college (David Baum). The tree is placed on a green field referring to Roy Meadow, the midwife of the College.

Coats of arms began in England in the Middle Ages, to distinguish individuals during tournaments. The knight carried his shield, distinctively painted, and wore his helmet with a crest. The idea was not original. In ancient times, Jewish, Greek and Roman families adopted special symbols. Armorial bearings are commonly called a coat of arms, but heraldically this term refers only to the devices borne on a shield. The full display of all the devices is called an achievement. The central element is the shield, which is surmounted by a helmet on which borne the crest. Mantling, representing protective drapery, flows from the helmet. The figures at the sides of the shield are called supporters.

Royal College of Paediatrics and Child Health

Coat of Arms

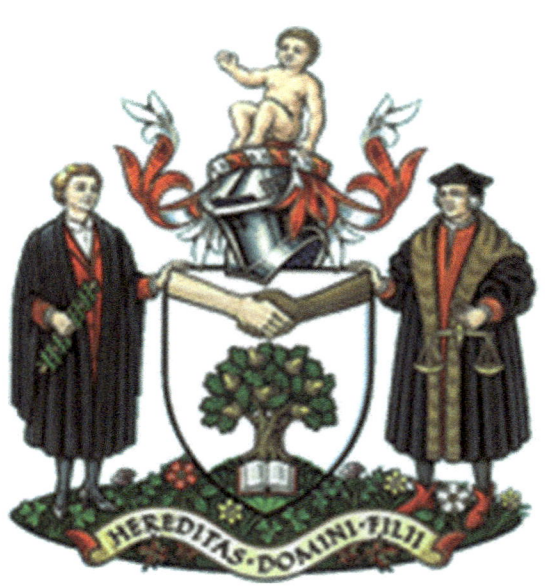

The Family

Right Supporter
Father figure of Thomas Phaire who was the author of the first book in English (1545) in contemporary academic dress. He is holding scales which signify the role of the College in setting standards and professional examinations.

Left Supporter
Mother figure with red hair in modern academic dress resembling Baroness Lloyd of Highbury who was the first woman President of the British Paediatric Association. She is holding a rod with a double-stranded helix indicating the importance of science, and in particular, genetics, to advances in child health.

This device also refers back to the serpent entwined staff of Aesculapius.

Crest
A child to represent the concept that the aspiration of parents and paediatricians should reach a level of attainment which is higher than their own. The child has been redrawn from the coat of arms of the Foundling Hospital at Coram Fields to show an association with children's hospitals.

The College

Shield
Oak tree on green meadow to represent child development and health. A book to indicate education and scholarship. Two hands shaking to represent friendship, which was one of the first rules of the British Paediatric Association.

Base
Meadow in the shape of a globe to signify the responsibility of the College towards children throughout the world. At the inaugural meeting of the British Paediatric Association, representatives of the different regions of the British Isles were appointed, and the College is still constituted in this democratic way as shown emblematically by the rose, the thistle, the shamrock and the daffodil. Maple leaves commemorate Donald Paterson who was the driving force for the inauguration of the British Paediatric Association and served as a leader for the first 20 years.

Motto
From Psalm 127. Hereditas Domini Filii. Children are a heritage of the Lord.

When David Baum became President, he appointed a small committee to determine the regalia and ceremonies that would be desirable and to commission and implement them. The Royal College of Physicians of London had offered a mace as a founding gift, and other wishes included an anthem set to music, a grace before meals, a presidential badge, a flag and an academic gown for the President. There was disagreement about the gown, and David Baum designed and paid for it personally. The flag was designed but never made.

The Mace

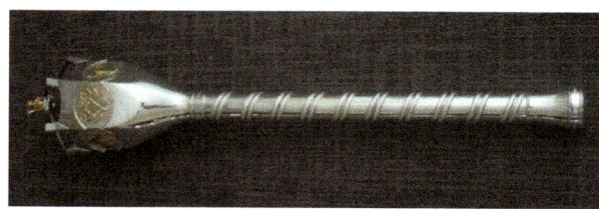

Mace

The mace was originally a weapon of combat and became a symbol of authority. Large numbers of ceremonial copper maces from the fourth millennium BC with a distinctive design have been found in the Near and Middle East. David Baum, President of the College and I, as Honorary Archivist, met the designer and silversmith Keith Hayman with the RCP Registrar, David London, and the RCP Secretary, David Lloyd, and the design was devised that day. The cost was £50,000. Keith Hayman, Fellow of the Institute of Professional Goldsmiths, has described the design.

'The mace is 1 m in length, was carved out of a solid block of metal and weighs 5.2 kg. The head of the mace is hexagonal and tapers into the round of the stem and is topped with a stylised crown, the arms of which bear the symbolic infant. Enclosed under the arms is a blue enamelled dome, upon which the coat of arms of the College, in full relief stands proud. The ring of stars of the European Union forms the border to the coat of arms and is set in the enamel, indicating the link the College has with the European Union. The hexagonal head of the mace provides six natural panels to accept six symbols: rose, daffodil, thistle, shamrock, maple leaf and scales. These emblems show that the College serves the whole of the British Isles, the first Honorary Secretary was Canadian and the College is responsible for setting standards.

At the base of the head is the engraved College motto: Hereditas Domini Filii. Around the polished stem is wrapped double helix, the stylized form of DNA strands. The butt of the mace is engraved with the coat of arms of the Royal College of Physicians of London who gave it'.

The mace was presented to David Baum, President of the Royal College of Paediatrics and Child Health, by George Alberti, President of the Royal College of

Physicians, on 15 July 1998 having ceremonially walked from the RCP in St Andrews Place a short distance away. David Baum considered that this gift was particularly appropriate because it symbolised the transfer of authority from the maternal ancient College to the infant College, after a gestation of 53 years and a difficult delivery, and of course it linked the new College back to 1518 and the Royal Charter granted by King Henry VIII.

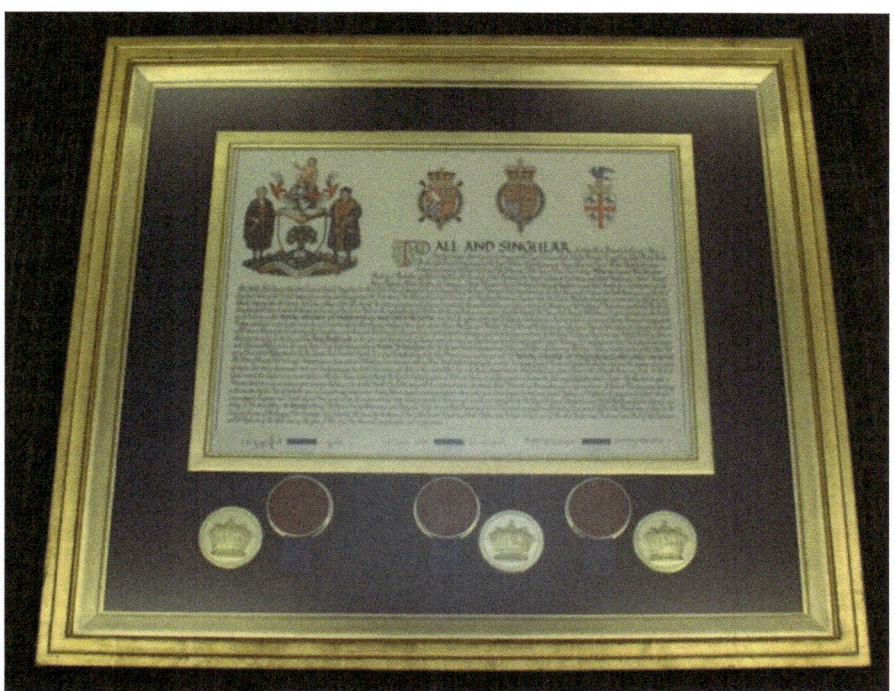

Royal Charter

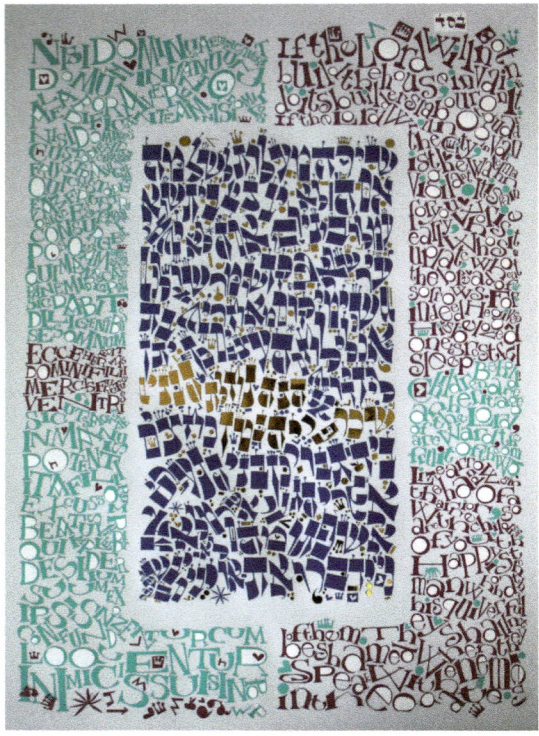

Scroll based on the College Psalm

The First Annual Meeting of the College 4

Andrew Wilkinson

Andrew Wilkinson, Professor of neonatology in Oxford, was the Chairman of the Academic Board when the college was founded and had overall responsibility for planning the first RCPCH Spring Meeting at York in 1997. His recollection of that memorable event follows.

Recollection of the First Annual Meeting of the RCPCH, University of York, 15–18 April 1997

The first Annual Meeting of the new college was held at York University in glorious spring weather. The daffodils were beautiful; the cherry blossom out in full, and the ducks and geese waddled everywhere on campus. The lake fountain was reaching its maximum height.

The format of the meeting was very much like the recent BPA meetings but there was an air of anticipation. This meeting really was going to be special and mark the beginning of a new era. Over 1500 paediatricians from the UK, Ireland and throughout the world had registered.

Special not least because our new patron, Her Royal Highness the Princess Royal, Princess Anne to most of us, was going to attend.

For Professor Sir Roy Meadow, who like Sir David Hull before him had done so much to lead the BPA into a Royal College, this was his last meeting as president, and he would hand over the reins to Professor David Baum at the Annual Dinner.

The scientific programme began with a brief history of the BPA and pages of archive photographs of the leaders of child health, with highlights of the achievements since the foundation in 1928.

A. Wilkinson
Oxford, UK

© Springer International Publishing Switzerland 2017
A. Craft, K. Dodd (eds.), *From an Association to a Royal College*,
DOI 10.1007/978-3-319-43582-4_4

43

On Wednesday, 16 of April, the Central Hall was searched with sniffer Alsatians prior to the arrival of the dignitaries. The red carpet was then road tested by a duck and her ducklings which were hurriedly shooed away by security men moments before the Princess Royal was due. All those attending the Special Plenary Session had to be seated 20 min before it began.

After four speakers, Princess Anne presented the certificates to new Honorary Fellows and the James Spence Medal to Barbara Ansell. She then addressed the audience for 15 min illustrating her passion for children's health throughout the world with examples of her experience as patron of *Save the Children*.

An informal buffet lunch followed with officers, staff of the college and the new Honorary Fellows.

Other celebrations of the founding of the college were to follow. The first AGM was held and after dinner was a question and answer session, chaired by the president, on *The Future of the College*.

On the evening of Thursday, 17 of April, instead of the traditional performance by the BPA orchestra, coaches left the University to take members to York Minster for a multifaith service of celebration. The weather continued to behave as a balmy breeze accompanied the participants who walked the last half mile to the Minster precincts.

As with the arrangements for the Royal Visit, the plans for the service had been thoroughly rehearsed. The Secretary of the Academic Board, Andrew Wilkinson, tirelessly assisted by the conference organiser Rosalind Topping and her assistant Amanda Ambalu, had agreed the plans with the Precentor, the Reverend Canon Paul Ferguson welcomed everyone of all faiths. The Girls of the Minster Choir, conducted by Philip Moore, sang and John Scott Whitley played the organ. The President, Roy Meadow, read a lesson, and the President-elect, David Baum, read Psalm 127 from which the motto of the new college derives – *Behold! Children are a heritage of the Lord*.

Following the service members made their way to York Racecourse where the Annual Dinner was held in the Ebor Room. To many people's surprise, the first speech '*To the College*' was given by the President of the RCP, Professor Sir Leslie Turnberg, who had voiced strong opposition to the creation of the college. He was generous in his congratulations and good wishes for the future relationship between the RCP and RCPCH. Professor Sir Roy Meadow replied and toasted the guests, and Professor Gavin Arneil, President of the International Paediatric Association, replied. The long-standing BPA Ulster Cup for squash and Schlesinger Dent Cup for golf were presented.

Apart from the excellent food, the highlight of the evening was a spectacular firework display watched from the fourth floor balcony of the racecourse stand. This lit up the sky over the racecourse. The company engaged to put on the fireworks had unfortunately overlooked the need to obtain permission from the police, and the noise alarmed many local residents! This led to the celebration of the foundation of the college reaching headline news, with photographs, in the morning newspapers!

Nevertheless the Scientific Meeting continued, and the high standard of presentation throughout the 4 days was a tribute to the investigators and many young speakers engaged in research into a wide range of child health issues.

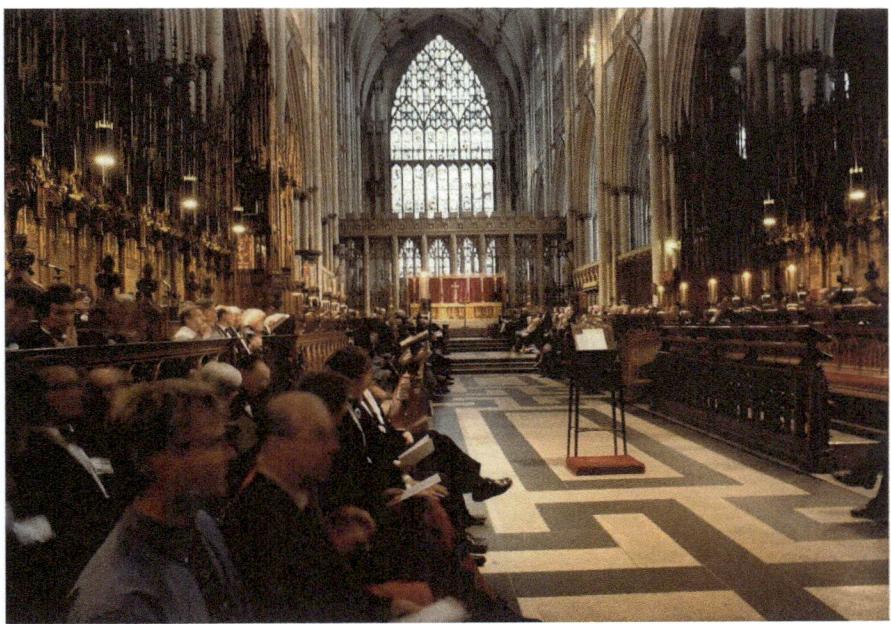

Inside York Minster at the multifaith service

Governance

5

Keith Dodd and Graham Sleight

Keith Dodd, who served as a senior College officer throughout the period covered by this history, describes the overnance of the BPA and the RCPCH and how it has, and still is, evolving. Graham Sleight who has been a senior staff member during this period adds his comments and brings the story up to date.

Keith Dodd Describes the Governance of the BPA and the RCPCH and How It Has, and Still Is, Evolving

The governance of the newly founded RCPCH was built on a large Council with a strong regional representative structure inherited from the BPA. Regional representation was based upon the prevailing NHS administrative structure of 21 Regional Health Authorities and Boards. The aim was to provide a democratic pathway for individual members via their regional representatives to Council. This generally worked well in Scotland, Wales and Northern Ireland, but only variably in the English regions, some of which had regular and formally constituted regional meetings, tagged on to educational events and supplemented when necessary by extraordinary meetings.

The decision to have a Council based on regional representatives had to be balanced by mechanisms to ensure the specialties were provided with a strong voice. The chosen route was initially through a Specialty Board with representatives on Council, and this was later strengthened by the formation of the College Specialty Advisory Committees (CSACs) which have, inter alia, major responsibilities for specialist training. In practice this worked well at Council level, whose members inevitably came from a wide range of specialties as well as generalists.

K. Dodd
Derby, UK

G. Sleight (✉)
London, UK

© Springer International Publishing Switzerland 2017
A. Craft, K. Dodd (eds.), *From an Association to a Royal College*,
DOI 10.1007/978-3-319-43582-4_5

Council is the college's ruling body, and its members are its trustees. It was supported by an Executive committee of college officers, which inevitably grew in size as the new responsibilities of the college expanded, including new roles such as ethics, advocacy, international affairs and the media. It soon numbered over 20. This in turn necessitated the formation of an informal President's Advisory Group, comprising senior officers meeting when necessary, and often frequently, mainly for the purpose of liaison but also to agree on division of work, priorities and action and the need for involvement of executive committee and Council.

Over the years it became evident that these governance structures had become unwieldy and needed to be reformed.

The important governance reforms agreed in 2016 should ensure a streamlined representative and democratic structure, supported by the dramatic improvements in communication over the last decade and in keeping with the needs of a modern college.

Governance Reforms

Graham Sleight, Head of Governance

The first page of Sir Thomas Malory's *Le Morte D'Arthur* – published in 1485 and set perhaps 1000 years earlier – mentions the college's regulators. According to Malory Uther Pendragon, the father of King Arthur found himself "desiring to have lain by" the wife of the Duke of Cornwall. But, being hampered in his desires, "then he called to him his Privy Council" and sought their advice. On this occasion, the Privy Council's advice proved unhelpful, so Uther Pendragon turned instead to Merlin. Merlin no longer being available, the RCPCH must seek advice from the same Privy Council. Members should be reassured, however, that most of our queries to them concern alterations in our governing documents.

In Chap. 2, the college's solicitor Bertie Leigh describes the work he undertook to establish the college's first Royal Charter and Bye-Laws, in collaboration with the President and Officers of the college in the mid-1990s. That set of governing documents created a structure for the college's governance that continued for almost 20 years. However, like all institutions, the college sometimes has to respond to pressures for change. A number of factors made the governance arrangements established in 1996 difficult to sustain by the mid-2010s.

In the first place, the Council – the Board of Trustees – set up in 1996 had, after subsequent modifications, a potential maximum of 51 members. It became increasingly clear that the sheer size of this group was an impediment to effective decision-making. Related to this was the issue that, as public-sector austerity tightened after the financial crash of 2008, it became more and more difficult for members to be released from their NHS Trust work to undertake roles as college trustees. Finally, as time passed and the complexity and reach of the college grew, so did the scale of the decisions that Council was asked to take. It became apparent that for a £16 M organisation, as the college was by this stage, specialist Trustees with professional experience of finance or legal issues might be needed – and such Trustees might not necessarily be members. Many of the other Medical Royal Colleges had dealt with similar challenges, and it was made clear that the RCPCH was not exempt from needing to consider these problems.

As Prof Ellis describes in her contribution to this book, a first attempt to reform the college's governance was made in autumn of 2014 (see Chap. 23). The president of the time, Dr Hilary Cass, had pursued with great energy a proposal to expand the college's structure to incorporate a multi-professional Foundation of Child Health. Changes to the governing documents presented to an EGM on 30 September 2014 would have established this Foundation while reforming the college's governance to address the challenges set out above. The EGM, held at the Institute of Education in London, saw strong views expressed on all sides, not least from those who remembered the struggle to establish the college described elsewhere in this book. In the end, the proposals received the approval of 54% of the 216 members who voted – less than the two-thirds majority required to enact them.

Dr Cass's successor, Prof Neena Modi, took office in the spring of 2015. Although she had not been in favour of the Foundation proposals, she was supportive of the need to deal with the problems of the 1996 governance structures. In a series of discussions early in Prof Modi's presidency, a new set of governance reforms were considered and ultimately agreed by Council in July 2015. The main features of these reforms were:

- A Board of Trustees comprising 12 members, including an independent chair, external experts on areas such as finance and charity law and a representative of children as the college's ultimate beneficiaries. A majority of the trustees will be college members, including the president, treasurer and registrar.
- A reformed Council comprising 21 members. This includes the President and other senior officers, members from geographical constituencies covering the whole of the UK and representatives of groups such as trainees and SAS doctors.
- A strengthened regional structure, with greater in-house support for members working in college roles across the UK.

Following that, the changes were drafted as alterations to the college's governing documents by Bertie Leigh's colleague Ian Hempseed. There then followed a lengthy series of discussions with the Privy Council to secure their approval. This was finally obtained in March 2016, and the changes were put before the AGM in Liverpool on 27 April 2016. For the first time, members were able to vote remotely by post or online in advance of the meeting. Very gratifyingly, the total turnout of voters was 1058, and 96% of them supported the changes.

At the time of writing (May 2016), with the AGM's approval achieved, work is now beginning on recruiting the new Trustees and other postholders required by this set of reforms. The important point to stress, however, is that the college's aims have not changed. The four objectives set out in the college's 1996 Royal Charter remain unchanged. The new challenge which these reforms present is to find ways to deliver those objectives in a health service environment which has changed radically – and doubtless will continue to change.

Interface with Government and Outside Bodies Including the Media

6

Alan Craft, Keith Dodd, Harvey Marcovitch, and Melissa Rome

The editors here describe the development of the College relationships with government, the NHS and other outside bodies. Links with the press have evolved over the years from a very informal reactive stance to one which is both reactive and very proactive.

Since the advent of the NHS in 1947, government has taken an increasing interest in health. Discussions with the medical profession around contractual issues are largely the province of the British Medical Association, and the BMA continues to be the trade union.

Advice to government has changed over the years. The Chief Medical Officer for many years had a special adviser in paediatrics, the last of these being David Hull who was the president of the BPA, but this formal arrangement is no longer in place. The CMO often does seek professional advice but more usually on an ad hoc basis around specific issues. Professor Liam Donaldson was much involved in public health issues, e.g. around safety and smoking rather than the delivery of care, but like his predecessor, Kenneth Calman, he was involved in trying to rationalise training, partly driven by the need to harmonise across Europe to enable free movement of labour. This is covered in the chapter on training. The latest CMO, Dame Sally Davies, has taken on specific themes and in 2012 children were her special area which formed the content of her annual report – 'Our Children Deserve Better;

A. Craft (✉)
Newcastle, UK

K. Dodd
Derby, UK

H. Marcovitch
Oxford, UK

M. Rome
London, UK

© Springer International Publishing Switzerland 2017
A. Craft, K. Dodd (eds.), *From an Association to a Royal College*,
DOI 10.1007/978-3-319-43582-4_6

Prevention Pays' – which was strongly supported by the RCPCH and to which many members and fellows contributed.

The Department of Health has employed paediatricians to work for them to provide input into strategy and advise on problems of the day. During the period covered by this volume, Drs Ian Lister Cheese and Roddy Mcfaul, Professor Al Aynsley Green and Dr Sheila Shribman have occupied this role, and currently Dr Jacquie Cornish is in post although since the latest NHS reforms in 2012 she has been employed by NHS England and any advice to DH has been sought on an ad hoc basis. Professor Stuart Tanner and Dr Ted Wozniak have worked within the DH bringing their knowledge of current paediatric issues to the centre where policy can be influenced. All of these paediatricians have worked with the BPA and RCPCH seeking advice when needed and working with the RCPCH to develop specific areas of work. Dr McFaul took a specific interest in policy and workforce development and the data which he collected on manpower was crucial in helping the rapid development of paediatrics as a specialty. Al Aynsley Green was appointed at a time when National Service Frameworks were the DH's mantra. The first on cancer, cardiology and mental health were accompanied by targets and substantial implementation money were very successful in improving outcomes for adults. However, by the time it came to that for children, 'Every Child Matters' which provided a comprehensive framework for the improvement of care for children, targets were no longer prescribed, and it was unfortunately not accompanied by money for implementation. These formed the basis of the cross-government policy of 'Every Child Matters' which has provided the important framework with which care has been developed in recent years. Another important organisational issue was that responsibility for questions around social care of children and issues such as safeguarding transferred from the Department of Health to the Department of Education. The RCPCH therefore needed to work with both of these Departments.

Throughout this period of the history of the BPA/RCPCH, we also had, in 1999, the devolution of power to the other three countries of the UK. This has meant the RCPCH works with four different governments and four slightly different versions of the NHS.

Before the advent of the RCPCH, most of any professional advice which was needed was obtained from the RCPCH, and indeed this was one of the main driving forces for the formation of a separate RCP. Successive presidents of the new College have found ways of working with ministers and civil servants in many government departments. There is no doubt that in 2016 the RCPCH is a major source of advice to government and indeed also helps to set policy and strategy. The DH Policy Advisers act as a bridge between government and the College, and although they generally do not have much in the way of a budget, they can often steer the College towards sources of funding which have helped initiatives develop when the College is best placed to pursue them. A good example of this is the Colleges' recent work on e-learning for disabled children. The College was seen as a body with status and one which was trusted and could deliver.

Another development over the last 15 years has been the establishment by government of 'arms length bodies'. There have been many of these with which the

College has had to interface including NICE (National Institute for Clinical Excellence) and the NPSA (National Patient Safety Agency).

The last 15 years have also seen the establishment of the role of Children's Commissioners in all four nations, and the College has needed to find ways of working with these. The College has recognised the importance of working with government and has been fortunate in the paediatricians who have devoted themselves within the Department of Health to work together for the benefit of children.

The Press

Harvey Marcovitch and Melissa Rome

The BPA and the RCPCH have always needed to respond to the press.

For many years Dr Harvey Marcovitch, a general paediatrician from Banbury, having been appointed as honorary editor of the BPA and editor of Archives of Disease in Childhood, found himself responsible for dealing with an increasing number of media enquiries. Mostly these were related to matters that had suddenly excited the attention of news desks, such as fabricated illness, unusual forms of child abuse, chronic fatigue syndrome and the (fraudulently) alleged association between immunisation and autism. Inevitably an instant response was requested which was generally best avoided whilst formulating a considered response. Insistent demands, especially to appear on broadcast media, led to developing a database of colleagues who would be prepared to respond to such demands.

Gradually, newspaper and broadcast media medical correspondents and feature writers started to make less fevered requests to help them make sure their articles were accurate. This included the editors of a popular BBCTV soap opera, Holby City, seeking paediatric approval of scripts for a time until new production values prioritised characters' personal relationships above medical verisimilitude.

Following the formation of the RCPCH, the increasing volume of press enquiries, as well as the need to work with the press to proactively get messages across, became clear. The College therefore appointed an experienced press officer to the staff, and over the years the College has worked well with the various aspects of the media and has gained a great deal of experience. Melissa Rome, who is the current head of media and external affairs, reflects on her time with the College along with comments from Harvey Marcovitch.

The RCPCH is in a prime position when it comes to securing media coverage. With its focus on babies and children, a bank of medical experts at its fingertips and the gravitas that comes with a royal charter, the College should be the 'go to' for comment on child health issues in the media and amongst key decision makers. But in order to be so, the College's resources – both in terms of its paediatrician members and its staff – need to be fully utilised.

When I applied for the post of Media and Campaign Manager at the RCPCH, I had already formed a view of its approach to media work. I suppose it was the 'royal' badge that made me assume it would be a largely conservative organisation, afraid to say anything too bold in the media for fear of offending the establishment and with a desire to communicate with the external world in formal, medically riddled language.

The reality was refreshingly different.

The RCPCH is unique amongst the medical royal colleges in that it doesn't solely represent its profession (i.e. it's not the Royal College of Paediatricians). The child health element means we enjoy a much broader remit – to campaign and drive policy change on key issues relating to child health.

Prior to staff being in place to deliver media and communications work for the College, the task fell to a dedicated RCPCH Council Member. Undoubtedly many health journalists would have been delighted to have the direct number of a paediatrician for comments and insights on their child health stories. But finding time to push out the College's messages to the media, promote College research and be proactive when it comes to media relations must have been a nigh on impossible task. So the decision to employ dedicated staff marked a real step forward for the College. We now have a small staff team working on media, public affairs and external affairs that work across the four nations of the UK.

Part of growing the RCPCH's media profile has centred around establishing a distinctive tone. The College must be authoritative and evidence based in what it says – a reliable and balanced voice when it comes to all things relating to child health. But crucially, evidence comes in the form not only of findings from research or medical studies (which is of course vital) but also the day-to-day experiences of doctors on the ground – their interactions with children, families and the wider health system. This has been the bedrock of media and campaigning work in the College in recent times, helping to move the RCPCH closer to being the 'go to' organisation on child health.

There are broadly three types of media work that we undertake: reactive, proactive and proactively reactive. With a small staff team dedicated to media, the challenge was to continue and expand the reactive work, increase the amount of proactive work (e.g. promoting the College's research and policy output) and build strong relationships with journalists, politicians, other charities and campaign organisations to make sure we are in a position to comment on child health media stories ahead of them being published (the so-called 'proactively reactive' work).

The strength of the College is its members and they are central to the RCPCH's media profile. Our ever-growing press panel now includes over 150 paediatricians from trainees to retired members, who are happy to speak to the media on behalf of the College. Some enjoy TV and radio work, and others are happy to give quotes to national or local newspapers, offer their expertise to child health magazines or blog on relevant websites. We are conscious of how busy members are and media involvement can be as little or as much as members want, and are able, to do.

We provide free media training for all RCPCH members who want it – a full day on using the media effectively with practice TV and radio interviews conducted by trained journalists. We run sessions in London, Cardiff, Glasgow and Belfast, which are always well attended, and feedback from members is hugely positive.

There have been numerous high-profile and challenging media stories involving the College, including the Health and Social Care Act (now Bill), the recent junior doctor contract negotiations and the thankfully relatively rare serious case reviews involving children.

In terms of our proactive work, in 2012 the College's policy and communications team led the Academy of Medical Royal College's obesity campaign – resulting in front page and widespread media coverage – and the establishment of an all-party parliamentary group on obesity. We've also run campaigns to highlight the dangers of vitamin D deficiency of children, to 'save the stats' when the Office for National Statistics threatened to stop publishing child mortality statistics and to raise the profile of the lack of funding for child health research. We have worked closely with other charities and campaign groups to lend our voice to successful campaigns such as the banning of smoking in cars with children present, standardised cigarette packaging and the UK's relatively poor child mortality rates. We work closely with the College's research team to promote the findings of audits on diabetes, epilepsy and neonates to a wide audience. Ahead of the UK 2015 general election and the elections in the devolved nations of the UK, we campaigned for the parties to make pledges to improve child health, and encouragingly, many of the manifestos included child health commitments.

It's often difficult to measure the success of the press and public affairs work. Whilst you can count individual pieces of coverage, it is meaningless unless the content is strong and the outlets are appropriate. Ultimately, the aim is to use the media coverage to generate positive policy change for child health. So when the Health Secretary announced the government would be publishing an obesity strategy, it was clear that tackling the nation's weight problem was finally being taken seriously at the highest levels. And something the College had been calling for – a tax on sugary drinks – has finally come to fruition.

Moving forward, we're looking to work more closely with children and young people to ensure their voices are reflected in the College's media work. We'll also continue to grow our social media profile, allowing us to engage with more members and link up with other organisations to campaign more effectively.

If there's one thing that's certain about media and external affairs work, it's that it never stands still. And so for the RCPCH to remain relevant and lead the way in child health, it has to be agile and continue to move with the times.

Melissa Rome
Head of Media and External Affairs

The Involvement of Children and Young People in the Work of the College

7

Emma Sparrow

Children and young people's right to participation is laid out in the United Nations Convention on the Rights of the Child (1989). Paediatricians have a duty to respect, protect and fulfil the rights of children. The UNCRC is based on the premise that children and young people have the same inherent worth as adults, should be afforded respect and are entitled to preservation of their dignity, whilst recognising the particular difficulties that children and young people face in influencing decision-making. The UNCRC establishes participation as a right for all children and young people and is not limited by age, social status, disability or other characteristic of the child or young person and that participation is voluntary and applies to all matters concerning the child or young person.

Article 12 states

> Parties shall assure to the child who is capable of forming his or her own views the right to express those views freely in all matters affecting the child, the views of the child being given due weight in accordance with the age and maturity of the child. For this purpose, the child shall in particular be provided the opportunity to be heard in any judicial and administrative proceedings affecting the child, either directly or through a representative or an appropriate body, in a manner consistent with the procedural rules of the nation.

This has clear links and synergy with the work of the College and the role of paediatricians to respect, protect and fulfil the rights of the child in relation to health.

The voice of children and young people within their healthcare is ever evolving, and hearing that voice is now seen as central to decision-making and essential to improving outcomes. Since its inception the Royal College has been committed to not only engaging patient and carer voices in informing and shaping their work and decisions and in understanding patient experience but has been increasingly

E. Sparrow
London, UK

© Springer International Publishing Switzerland 2017
A. Craft, K. Dodd (eds.), *From an Association to a Royal College*,
DOI 10.1007/978-3-319-43582-4_7

recognised as championing the voice of children and young people. Visitors to the College will see the children and young people's presence and views proudly displayed on the walls through artwork created to celebrate the tenth birthday which shows the difference paediatricians make every day to the lives of children, young people and their families.

Children's drawings/paintings

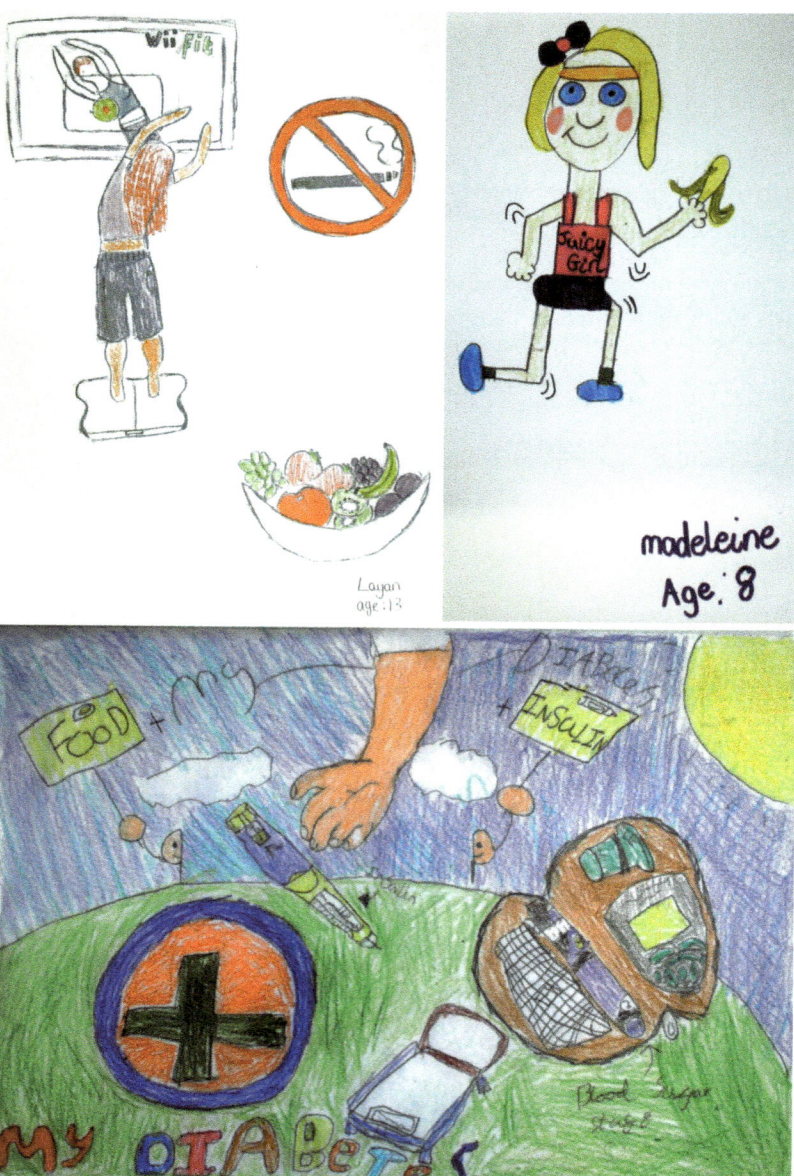

Over the years there have been a number of different models tried and tested for engaging the voice of children, young people and their families in shaping policy and practice in both the College and child health. In the early part of the twenty-first century, a patient and carer committee was established providing scope and remit for a strategic voice to become embedded. A number of dedicated and committed parents and carers regularly met with senior and junior officers and members of staff at all levels to inform and influence research, publications, audit work and training and assessment of trainees. In 2007, the move to directly involve young people was strengthened with the formation of the first Youth Advisory Panel. The panel brought together a small group of young people to discuss priorities for child health and to identify potential solutions and platforms for sharing the views of children and young people strategically. Young people who were part of the Youth Advisory Panel travelled across the UK, speaking about obesity in Westminster and child health debates in Scotland and Northern Ireland, participating in conferences on "My Right to the Highest Standard of Health in Wales, supporting the development of Patient Reported Experience Measure (PREM) tools", supporting the writing of National Institute for Health and Care Excellence (NICE) guidelines on transition, inputting into the Chief Medical Officer's annual report and more.

In keeping with the College's commitment to children's rights, in December 2010, the College hosted an interactive and stimulating training event exploring how the United Nations Convention on the Rights of the Child (UNCRC) is relevant to paediatrics, the College and its committees. In 2009, the College also marked the 20th anniversary of the United Nations Convention on the Rights of the Child. Guest speakers included Alex Willsher (RCPCH Youth Advisory Panel Member) and Sir Al Aynsley Green (Children's Commissioner for England).

Young people and families have been a feature of the College Spring Meeting and Annual Conference for a number of years, with members of the Youth Advisory Panel opening the conference with the President. They have continued sharing their views through plenary sessions and workshops on rights, engagement and patient experience. In addition to supporting College conference activity, children, young people and their families have been at the heart of key College and Consortia projects such as MindEd, Disability Matters, MedsIQ, Medicines for Children and more.

The College has created a number of publications with children, young people and their families over the years to support their voice in making a difference. Notably the "Not Just a Phase" report with the Young People's Health Special Interest Group published in 2010 provided guidance for paediatricians starting on their journey of participation and engagement. With a theoretical context and practical tools, it became a key feature in the recent development of children and young people's voices in child health and healthcare. Building on the learning from the report and Turning the Tide in 2012, the College launched Research & Us® in 2016, an Infants', Children's and Young People's Child Health Research Charter with a "what you need to know" guide and useful links and resources download.

Recent developments see children and young people's voice at the centre of the College strategic plan under "Inform, Child Rights, Influence". The establishment of the & Us® Network in 2015 moved the model for children, young people and family engagement on to a virtual network with greater reach and scope. Since January 2016, over 220 children and young people have actively commented on child health policy, shared their view and supported training and raising awareness of patient experience in child health and healthcare. In 2016, a practitioner network was launched called the Engagement Collaborative, providing resources and opportunities to discuss strategic voices at a professional network level.

Emma Sparrow

Children and Young People's Engagement Manager

Finance

8

John Osborne

Professor John Osborne, a general paediatrician in Bath, and Treasurer, engineered the complex transition from an association with a simple financial structure to a college with responsibility for education, training and examinations. These functions, previously managed by the 'ancient' colleges but largely run by paediatricians, were the subject of difficult and potentially hazardous negotiations, as John's account demonstrates.

Finance

The years before the formation of our college were, from a financial point of view, the lull before the storm. However, they were anything but dull, and the actions taken by my predecessors were essential to the satisfactory position the British Paediatric Association (BPA) was in financially whilst the negotiations were taking place. With just under £1 million in reserves when we became a College, we were not in a position of plenty, but the persistence of Christopher Nourse in successfully obtaining a VAT refund of £100,000 and an improvement in our investments of £60,000 through careful management were significant and essential benefits. For the BPA, the main sources of income were the annual meeting, member's subscriptions, grants and income from the Archives of Disease in Childhood. However, it was clear that a substantial increase in income would be required to take on the vital key roles of a College – training and examinations.

The negotiation for the transfer of the paediatric examination for membership to the new Royal College of Paediatrics and Child Health (RCPCH) was a complex affair not made any easier by having to negotiate with three Colleges of Physicians – London, Edinburgh and Glasgow (the latter a College of Physicians and Surgeons) – who jointly ran the membership of the Royal Colleges of Physicians MRCP (UK) examination, coordinated through the MRCP office based in London and run by

J. Osborne
Bath, UK

© Springer International Publishing Switzerland 2017
A. Craft, K. Dodd (eds.), *From an Association to a Royal College*,
DOI 10.1007/978-3-319-43582-4_8

the London College on behalf of all three Colleges. Their senior officers met officially about three times per year, and it was at these meetings that high-level discussions would take place. The President of our new College was invited to these meetings and usually asked the President-elect, David Baum, and myself to attend. They were very formal and to my mind very boring with each side jockeying for position and unwilling to give anything away – especially if it had a financial impact. Decisions rarely seemed to be made. The underlying view at these meetings was that the examinations were an asset that belonged to the three Colleges and which should be bought. The opposing view, led by myself, was that the examinations, and in particular the questions, were the intellectual property of paediatricians and that to withhold them would be a very aggressive act. I pointed out that they risked a wholesale resignation of paediatric members and fellows from their Colleges. However, the stumbling block remained that the presidents would discuss these issues briefly before deciding to ask the three treasurers to negotiate the transfer – but without giving them any guidance on which to base the transfer.

Whilst the preliminary discussions were taking place, plans were made to set up an examination of our own: not only did this seem wise, but it would help to strengthen our negotiating hand. There was, once a year, a meeting of clinical tutors to keep them up to date with the rapidly changing training environment at the time. With the agreement of Graham Clayden, the head of examinations for the paediatric MRCP, I wrote to each tutor and asked them to bring with them five possible questions for a new part 1 examination. At the end of the day, we had collected 200 multiple choice questions – only needing 60 for a part 1 paper!

In addition, David Baum visited Australia and came back with an offer to allow us to use the whole of their paediatric question bank – a very generous and helpful offer. This forward planning proved to be worth its weight in gold. Graham Clayden was a great help, making it clear that in his view, the questions belonged to the paediatricians who had helped develop them and that they, not the Colleges, owned the copyright. This was the only unambiguous help from a key paediatrician within the London College and the MRCP office. Others had been heard to say they thought it was only fair that we should agree to pay £1 million for the examination – more than the assets of the BPA. I had to make it very clear to them that whilst I was treasurer, we would not be paying to take over the paediatric examination.

However, I was delighted to read that the three Royal Colleges running the MRCP (UK) had decided that anyone who had entered the examination should be allowed to finish and be awarded the MRCP (UK). This statement was published in the BMJ soon after we became a College, and it pointed out that candidates who had started the examination had 7 years in which to finish it – thus committing the ancient Colleges to running a paediatric clinical examination until the end of 2003. I believe the ancient Colleges thought that this was a clever move on their part, protecting their income from the paediatric examination for some years to come, but it played right into our hands.

I was forever being told that running the examination was very difficult with the implication that our new College would not be able to do this without all the help of the MRCP office – for which they would charge. I found this difficult to believe – an opinion that was confirmed when in January 1997, we found that the MRCP office had failed to recruit sufficient clinical sites for the paediatric examination in February. They had written to the candidates but had not had the courtesy to inform our College – this did after all affect our trainees, not theirs, whoever was organising the examination. With only 6 weeks to go to the date of the clinical examination, I managed to organise 3 days of examination at my hospital in Bath. This was not as impossible as I had been told but was run without incident and had the effect of showing those in our College, as well as those in the ancient Colleges, that we could run a clinical examination without any real difficulty. At the time I was a Diploma of Child Health (DCH) examiner but not an MRCP examiner, which I was told would make it impossible for Bath to run the examination. However, it was the support of my colleagues in Bath that made this possible. They, like paediatricians elsewhere, were both strongly supportive of the new College and were very disappointed at the lack of support for paediatrics shown by the London College and the MRCP office.

Running the MRCP paediatrics overseas was frequently being mentioned as another area where we would be unable to run the examination without the help of the MRCP office. It was complex – with different agreements in different countries for different parts of the examination – part 1, part 2 and the clinical. The agreements at each site also ran for different periods of time. In order to keep on top of this and other issues, I read and made notes on the examination regulations and the overseas memoranda of understanding (MOUs) between the UK Colleges and sites overseas. This helped us to write our own examination regulations in preparation for the take over and also gave me valuable insight that often allowed me to negotiate around difficulties in the months ahead.

Thus came the day when, for the second time, a meeting of the Treasurers of the three ancient Colleges was asked by their Presidents to agree a financial deal to hand over the paediatric MRCP examination. The first meeting had concluded that the Treasurers could not make a decision until the Presidents gave them more specific guidance. I was invited to 'attend' these meetings but on the second occasion was given my head by David Baum to do the best I could to finalise a deal, with the promise that he would support whatever I could agree. What the Treasurers did not know was that we had also agreed that the procrastination could not continue: if we could not agree a transfer, then we would set up our own examination. The meeting began and yet again came to the initial conclusion that no decision could be made unless we agreed to pay £1 million. I then stated that we would have to set up our own examination as we could no longer wait for an agreement, and I explained the preparations we had made, with question banks and clinical sites already in place. I then asked how they expected to run a clinical examination for their remaining MRCP candidates – given that it would only take one consultant at each site to refuse to help hold a paediatric examination for the MRCP examination to make it impossible to do so. However, if they handed over the examination, including question banks, without charge, then we would agree to examine the remaining paediatric MRCP candidates on their behalf – splitting costs in proportion to the number of candidates for each examination, MRCP or MRCPCH. I well remember looking up to find three pale-faced shocked Treasurers looking at me! They had not seen this coming. After a short deliberation whilst I waited outside, I was asked in again and told that they agreed! I was delighted of course and remember telling them that I would set an example in thanks by publically stating that I would continue my FRCP of the London College at least until the end of the joint examination at the end of 2003. We agreed that each side would pay their share of costs with the exact timing of transfer of administrative arrangements being as soon as possible – the MRCP office needed more space! I was very amused and not a little proud to receive a Christmas card next December from the Treasurer of the London College – which was addressed 'to a worthy adversary'!

Initially we agreed that the overseas examinations would continue to be run by the MRCP office, since these were less important in laying down a marker of our College's independence than the UK examination. However, it was not so long before we were asked to take this over. In the interim, I had been able to visit most of the overseas clinical centres as an examiner in order to negotiate new MOUs with the organisations hosting the examination overseas.

Once the transfer of the membership examination was agreed, it was much easier to negotiate the transfer of the London DCH which was run by the London College. There was no problem of candidates who had already started the examination since, at that time, the written and clinical both had to be passed at the same sitting. We thus agreed that the RCPCH would take over the examination as soon as possible but, as a gesture of goodwill, the RCPCH would give to the RCP London half the surplus, if any, from the first year's two diets. I just had to make sure that we found as many costs as we could that year! But it must be remembered that examinations, whilst expensive for the candidates, are extremely expensive for Colleges to run, so finding costs was not difficult.

Accommodation

The BPA was housed at No. 5 St Andrews Place when news of its transmutation into a College was received. It had been an excellent home, provided by the RCP (L) at a peppercorn rent due to a charitable donation towards its refurbishment organised by a paediatrician, Prof. Sir Eric Stroud. The accommodation had already been outgrown with storage space being borrowed next door and many rooms being far too small for their purpose. A committee was formed to look for new accommodation and supported by the finance committee; I made it quite clear that we would only purchase a freehold property – not always an easy undertaking in London – but one which in the long term was clearly the only sensible way to go. My argument was supported by the simple statement that no one in their right mind would buy a leasehold property for their own money for their own residence, unless perhaps it was for 999 years.

After viewing several properties through an agent working on our behalf, none of which had a lay out or character suitable for a new College; we found that the Medical Protection Society (MPS) was selling their Hallam Street property. It seemed ideal and a purchase was made. A typical 1920s building, it had a metal frame that could be prone to rust if water ingress occurred, but there was no sign of that, and even the Empire State Building, built even earlier and in the same way, was still standing. A careful review of our likely needs suggested that the building should be big enough for about 5 years but not more than 10 years – a remarkably accurate prediction as it turned out. The day we took ownership, we asked our agent to find out who owned the freehold of all the buildings surrounding us and to our dismay discovered that the freehold of the matching building next door, rented by the GMC, had just been sold. For some time, we still hoped to be able to rent this as the GMC was considering relocation, but this never happened. We managed to convince the RCP London that we should retain the lease of No. 5 St Andrews Place to take into account future expansion – in particular for examinations – sufficiently well that we were then able to negotiate a donation of £100,000 to give up this space when we did move. Hallam Street proved a very suitable building with a council chamber large enough for membership ceremonies and even small academic meetings. We furnished it with sustainably sourced wood tables and chairs, and the Medical Protection Society kindly gave us the President's chair. The windows were draught-proofed to deaden sound from the street and a carpet was woven with our College crest – at no increased cost over providing the needed new carpet – and a College council chamber with suitable dignity was ours.

Funding from the Department of Health

At this time, several functions were required of Colleges in order to support the National Health Service (NHS) and were thus funded by the Department of Health. These included higher specialist training (HST), general professional training (GPT) and the overseas doctors training scheme (ODTS). These activities were carried out all over the UK, but the London College only ran those in England. Again it was made quite clear to us that they would not willingly hand over to us any of their NHS grant for these activities. We therefore negotiated directly with the NHS, quite reasonably making it clear that we could not commence these activities without the usual financial support. When it came to the next financial year, starting April 2007, we were given our full grant request and set about recruiting staff: I was led to believe that the funding was released by freezing for 1 year, the grants to other Colleges; whether all or just the London College, I never knew. This was the last major hurdle to our financial independence and security.

Summary

Thus we arrived, by the end of 1997, at the very satisfactory position of being secure in our new home and able to run the functions of a College without the need to significantly increase membership fees – as many opposed to the formation of our new College had predicted – and soon after were in charge of our own examinations. We had kept a very tight control of spending during this period, out of necessity, but that too meant that we were a lean organisation well prepared for the expansion that was to come. Even before the examinations were taken over, our assets had more than doubled. But then, as predicted, the membership of the new College increased rapidly as those passing the paediatric MRCP or the MRCPCH were entitled to become members. Unlike the three ancient Colleges, we made our successful candidate members of our College without further charge for the first year after their examination success. Those already awarded the MRCP (UK) in paediatrics, or in adult medicine if able to show that they worked in paediatrics, could also apply for membership of the RCPCH. There were just under 4,000 members of the BPA when we became a College, but this figure rose rapidly and was over 10,000 by the end of 2008. Whilst examination income also rapidly increased, the cost associated with running the examinations, and especially in revamping the examination to the new format more suitable for paediatrics, was very high but very necessary. This income peaked in 2005–2006 before falling due to reduced numbers taking the examination due to new rules affecting those from overseas wishing to train in the UK.

The Medicines for Children initiative, started by Sir David Hull, led to a steady income stream which was considerably enhanced with the development of this publication into the British National Formulary for Children (see later chapter). The other main factors affecting the financial stability of the new College was the revaluation of the Hallam street premises prior to the purchase of the current accommodation in Theobald's Road (the sale of Hallam Street raised £5.15 million more than it had cost), a legacy from one of our fellows that amounted to more than £1 million, the donation of £500,000 from Children Nationwide and the appeal in 1997 to members and fellows which raised over £100,000 – a highly significant sum at the time – being nearly 10% of our assets on formation of the College. The year 2008 found the College well established financially in our new home in Theobald's Road with a secure financial future and assets of nearly £18 million compared to £1.223 million at the time of formation of the College. The figures below indicate our growth in membership and assets and also where we currently receive our money from and where we spend it.

The following figures show the growth of the College assets and membership:

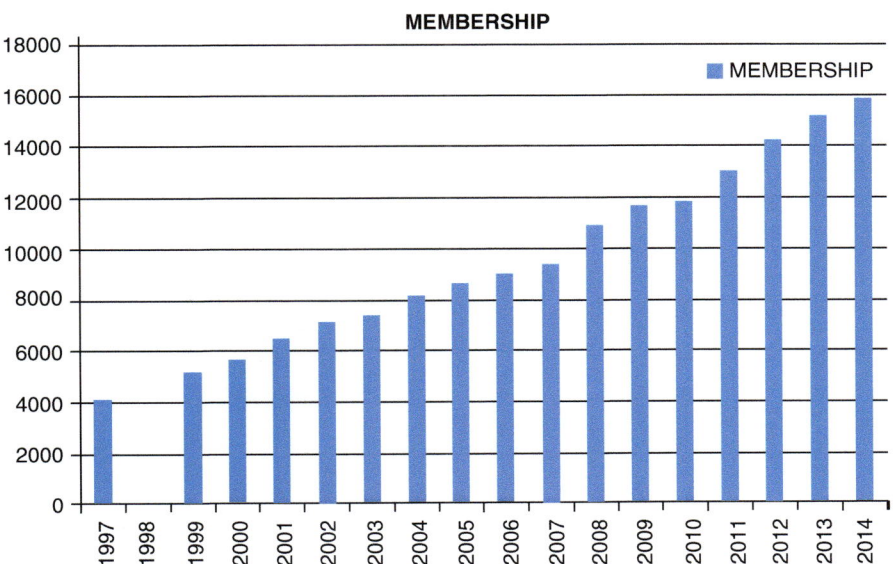

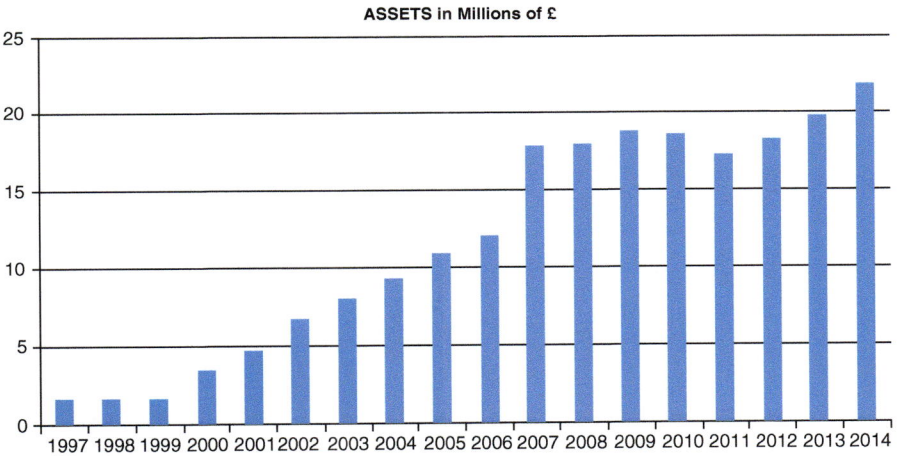

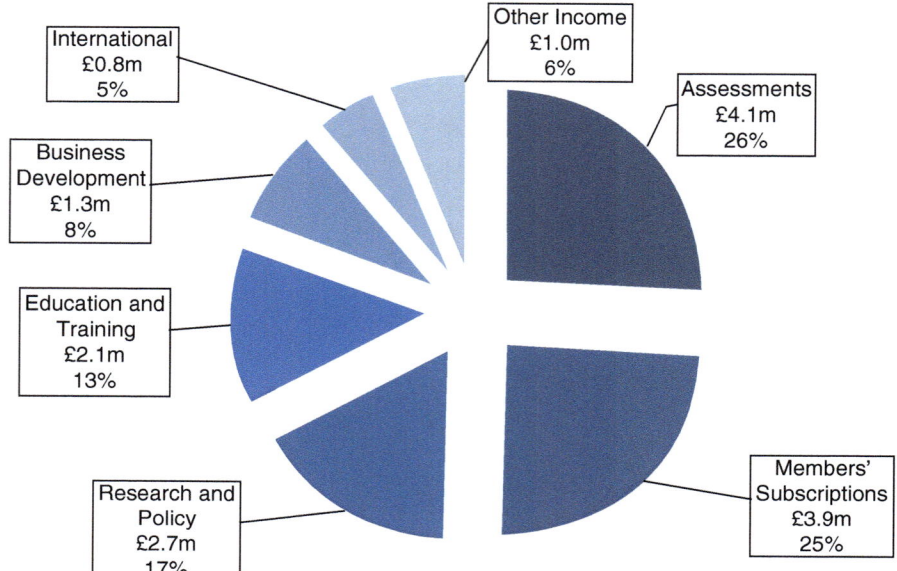

Income Summary 2014/15
Total=£15.9m

International £0.8m 5%

Other Income £1.0m 6%

Assessments £4.1m 26%

Business Development £1.3m 8%

Education and Training £2.1m 13%

Members' Subscriptions £3.9m 25%

Research and Policy £2.7m 17%

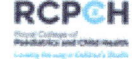

Expenditure 2014/15
Total=£16.1m

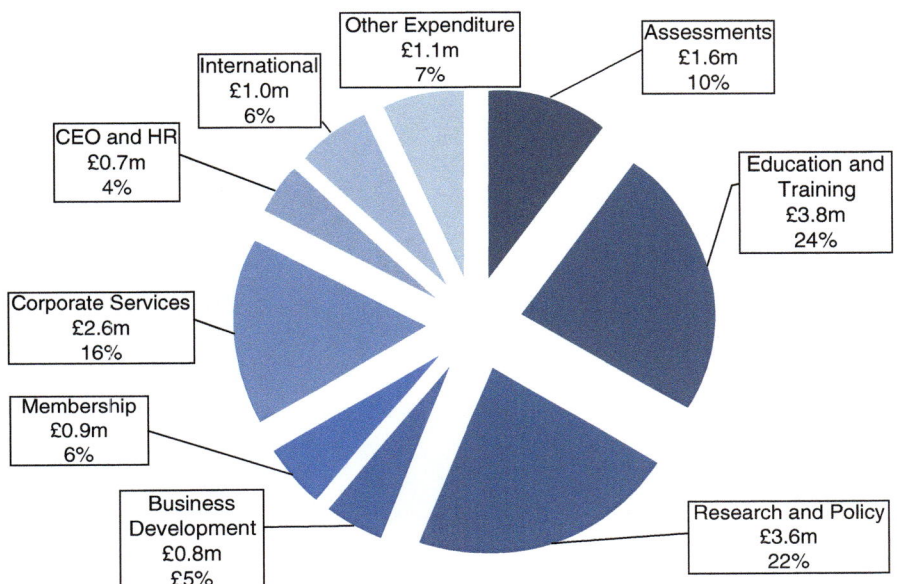

Other Expenditure
£1.1m
7%

International
£1.0m
6%

CEO and HR
£0.7m
4%

Corporate Services
£2.6m
16%

Membership
£0.9m
6%

Business
Development
£0.8m
£5%

Assessments
£1.6m
10%

Education and
Training
£3.8m
24%

Research and Policy
£3.6m
22%

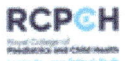

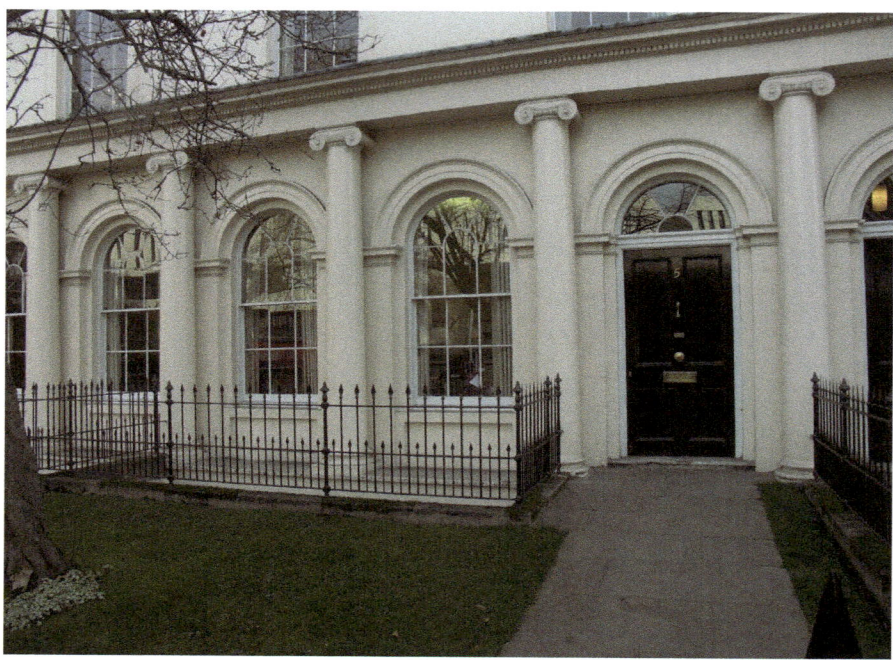

The College at St Andrew's Place

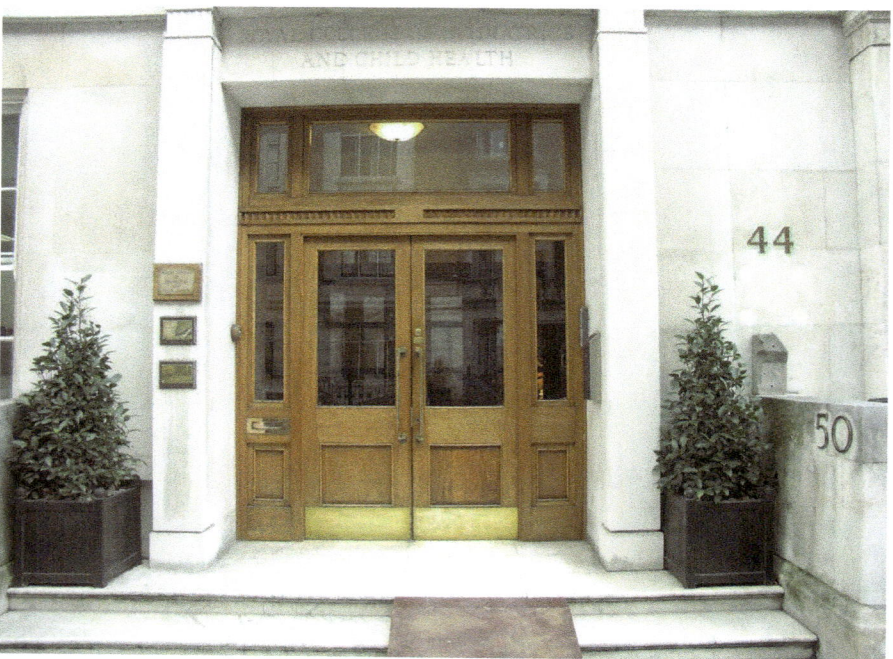

The College at Hallam Street

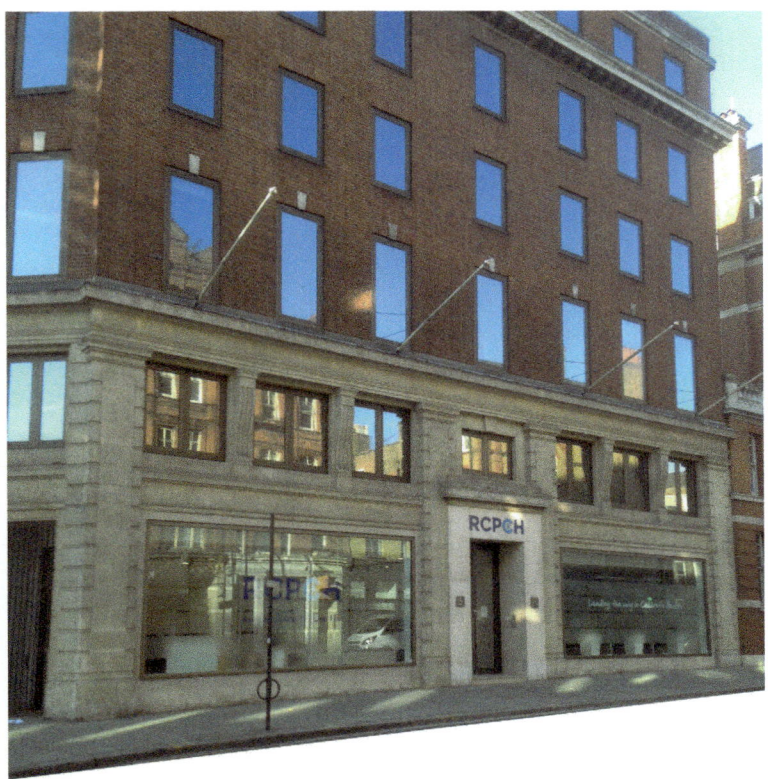

The College at Theobalds Road

Exams

9

Thomas Lissauer

While the financial negotiations over the new college were difficult, its success was predicted upon the successful running of the postgraduate examinations – many thought the project would fail. Graham Clayden and Tom Lissauer had already been actively involved in the exams, and their close and harmonious working relationship secured the success of the new Royal College of Paediatrics and Child Health (RCPCH) examinations. They adapted and developed it, introducing new formats, especially in the clinical parts of the exam, and underpinning this with careful training and monitoring of the examiners and audit of the exams process.

As maintaining the standards of doctors is a key function of Medical Royal Colleges, examinations play a pivotal role within the Royal Colleges, and establishing our independent examinations was a priority when the RCPCH was established.

The detailed negotiation of transfer of the exams has been well described by the College's first treasurer, John Osborne.

Before the 1970s, doctors wishing to become paediatricians had to pass the membership of the Royal Colleges of Physicians (MRCP) examination in adult medicine, with just a few questions of the written paper on children's illnesses. From 1972, candidates could take a paediatric option, which allowed them to answer a part of the written exam (Part 2 paper) and the entire oral and clinical exam in paediatrics and child health. Over the following 20 years, there was lively debate at the examination boards of the Royal Colleges of Physicians (RCP) in the UK about the increasing demand from trainees for a paediatric option of the first part of the MRCP (Part 1 paper). This was a 60 multiple true/false computer-marked paper of which only five questions covered child health subjects. A single paediatrician contributed to the MRCP Part 1 Examination Board, who frustratingly had to avoid paediatric-orientated questions that were

T. Lissauer
London, UK

© Springer International Publishing Switzerland 2017
A. Craft, K. Dodd (eds.), *From an Association to a Royal College*,
DOI 10.1007/978-3-319-43582-4_9

very relevant for paediatric trainees but not for those in general medicine. These subjects included topics such as child development, clinical embryology, basic paediatric surgery and immunisations. It was considered that the Diploma of Child Health covered such topics, but this exam was optional for trainees and only a minority took it.

During this time, paediatricians were represented on the council of the RCP (London) by the paediatric censor, although the arrangements in the two Scottish colleges were different. The MRCP (UK) was a jointly owned and organised examination by the three Royal Colleges of Physicians, and any attempts to alter the structure involved multiple and highly diplomatic engagement with three ancient college councils. A particular problem for paediatricians was that they were taking longer to pass MRCP (UK) Part 1 than their adult medicine colleagues.

Professor Dame June Lloyd, the paediatric censor of the RCPL at the time, managed to persuade the RCPs of the UK to hold a joint working party with the British Paediatric Association (BPA) about creating a paediatric option for the Part 1 exam. She chaired this committee, and by 1993, the first paediatric MRCP (UK) Part 1 took place, with 50 % overlap of questions with general medicine and the remainder covering the clinical science and practice of importance to paediatricians. This working party was the first official link between the RCPs and BPA and was an early forerunner of the creation of the RCPCH.

Following the formation of the RCPCH, the handover of the paediatric exams was gradually orchestrated. There were many sensitivities at the RCPs, and a number of paediatricians had to straddle the wide gulf between the parties. Key issues included the rights of candidates to complete the exams that they originally started with the ancient colleges, the considerable financial consequences for the ancient Colleges of transferring the exams and the copyright status of the exam question banks. These and many other difficult issues were dealt with by a planned partnership followed by slow withdrawal of the RCPCH from the MRCP (UK). This was orchestrated by Graham Clayden, who held the position of the last paediatric censor of the RCP (L), Chair of the Membership of Royal College of Paediatrics and Child Health (MRCPCH) Part 1 Examination Board and then the founding Officer for Examinations in the RCPCH in 1999. In view of the fact that the paediatric option of MRCP (UK) needed to be available for candidates for 7 years, the transfer of MRCPCH Part 2 was much slower. This gave Tom Lissauer, who was the Chairman of the MRCPCH/MRCP (UK) Part 2 Paediatric Examination and a member of the Policy Committee of the MRCP (UK), the benefit of being involved with the redesign of the MRCP (UK) Part 2 Clinical Examination in adult medicine. This greatly assisted him in setting up the new MRCPCH Part 2 exams for the RCPCH when he became the RCPCH Officer for Examinations in 2003. It also enabled him to organise the smooth transfer of examinations conducted overseas to the RCPCH.

The foundation of the RCPCH allowed a number of problems for paediatricians of the MRCP (UK) to be addressed. One of the driving factors in establishing the

RCPCH was the feeling that the formal control of the discipline of paediatrics in the UK was too focused on London and to a lesser degree, Edinburgh and Glasgow. The new MRCPCH Examination Board was deliberately based on wide regional representation through the establishment of the system of Principal Regional Examiners (PREs). Many of them were experienced MRCP examiners and created local question writing groups and also recruited local examiners to host the clinical exam in hospitals within their region. They, with representatives from Hong Kong and Singapore (where the RCPCH conducted the exams), formed the new RCPCH examination boards.

As the RCPCH gained control over the paediatric postgraduate exams, a more detailed training curriculum was compiled, and the exams were gradually restructured. It was clear that the Part 1 exam needed to split into two sections: Part 1a with questions on the range of clinical conditions that were most likely encountered by trainees in their first year and Part 1b focusing on the basic clinical sciences that underpinned paediatric practice. Success in Part 1a also allowed trainees wanting an additional qualification in paediatrics but not planning to become paediatricians to enter the Diploma in Child Health (DCH), creating a more streamlined approach to the paediatric examinations.

Under Dr Tom Lissauer's leadership, the clinical MRCPCH Part 2 examination was also radically transformed from the traditional long and short cases and viva to a ten-station examination with two communication and one history taking and management planning stations, five clinical stations (cardiovascular, respiratory, abdomen, musculoskeletal, neurological/neurodisability), child development and a station based on video scenarios. The video station incorporated the assessment of acute illness into the examination. An important innovation was to have only one examiner per station. After extensive piloting and intensive examiner training, the new clinical exam was successfully introduced.

Subsequent Officers for Examinations, Drs Simon Newell, Kevin Windebank and Jane Valente, have continued to develop the examinations. The written examinations have been changed from norm to criterion referenced to determine the pass mark, and new regulations around the exam have been steadily simplified.

New clinical examination centres have been developed overseas, including Egypt, India and Myanmar. None of these changes would have been possible without the creation of an excellent administrative team within the College. The current paediatric membership examination has been significantly changed and consists of the following three papers: Foundation of Practice (FOP), Theory and Science (TAS) and Applied Knowledge and Practice (AKP). Computer-based testing was successfully introduced both in the UK and at Overseas (OS) centres for the three theory papers in 2015.

To obtain the MRCPCH qualification, this is then followed by a clinical membership examination which consists of ten clinical stations as described above.

For those sitting the clinical Diploma of Child Health, the Foundation of Practice (FOP) theoretical paper common to both examinations needs to be passed first followed by the clinical DCH examination. The International DCH was introduced in 2015 in India.

The assurance that examiners provide a consistently applied method of clinical examination has always been a principle of the MRCPCH and DCH exams. Since 2011, there has been a robust application, selection and training process for new clinical examiners supported by experienced examiner trainers and the College exams team. This provides regional training and is transported overseas for new examiner training sessions there. In 2016, a Senior Examiner Training Course was introduced providing specific support for those experienced examiners recommended either to provide quality assurance during the UK diets or become an overseas examiner.

In 2015, 30 centres held the UK clinical examination, providing places for 1017 candidates.

By 2015, the MRCPCH/DCH theory examinations (FOP/TAS/AKP) ran in 17 countries with the MRCPCH Clinical being hosted in nine countries. During the course of this year, moves were being made to introduce the DCH exam in both Egypt and India.

It became evident during the introduction of new overseas centres that significant training for both hosting examiners and local candidates would be required. This was implemented by the PREs and the newly appointed Strategic Leads for the regions and delivered by the UK exam teams at each diet overseas. By 2016, most overseas exam diets now involve such training, at least 2 days of examinations and not infrequently locally delivered Continuing Professional Development (CPD) sessions.

The RCPCH is currently in the process of discussion with our overseas partners to ensure that the exam is appropriate with their training. Alongside overseas examining other continuing professional developments and training courses are held internationally. In 2016, the strategy for overseas exams was being closely reviewed by the newly formed International Education Board (IEB) which replaced the Overseas Exams Board. Assurance of relevancy and sustainability for the MRCPCH exam in relation to an overseas country were important key factors for the IEB.

The RCPCH has developed a comprehensive psychometric team who analyse and generate all examination pass marks and results, including undertaking rigorous quality checks, and perform post hoc statistical analysis on this data.

The Angoff method, a robust and established criterion-referenced approach, is used to set the standard (pass mark) for all theory examinations. This was introduced to the AKP exam in 2007 and to the FOP and TAS exams in 2012, in a move away from the norm-referenced Hofstee method.

Average pass mark and pass rate data for the three 2015 diets for the MRCPCH examinations are presented below.

Average data for 2015 exams	FOP exam (Foundation of Practice)	TAS exam (Theory and Science)	AKP exam (Applied Knowledge in Practice)	MRCPCH UK Clinical exam
Pass mark	62.86%	58.63%	59.73%	100/120
Pass rate – overall	50%	46%	55%	56%
Pass rate – UK graduates	72%	77%	70%	74%
Pass rate – OS graduates	40%	42%	50%	32%
Reliability (alpha)	0.82	0.84	0.76	0.61
SEM (standard error of measurement)	4.22	4.21	3.90	n/a

FOP, TAS and AKP Pass Mark Information

The pass marks for the Foundation of Practice, Theory and Science and Applied Knowledge in Practice examinations are criterion referenced using Modified Angoff methodology. Each candidate is judged against an absolute standard rather than relative to other candidates.

After the exams are held, a panel of professional judges independently grade each item of the exam and estimate the percentage of borderline candidates (the candidates who have a 50% chance of passing the exam) that will answer the question correctly. At the Angoff meeting, the individual judgements are displayed, and the panel discuss them before each judge scores again. The candidates' performance in the actual exam is then revealed, and the judges give final estimates, which when averaged becomes the final criterion-referenced score for the question. The weighted mean of all these final scores becomes the pass mark for the exam.

The performance of the exam questions is also assessed during this meeting; any questions that do not perform well are fully reviewed.

MRCPCH Clinical Examination Pass Mark Information

In total there are ten clinical stations, and the following marks will be awarded for each of the overall station judgements:

Clear pass – 12
Pass – 10
Bare fail – 8
Clear fail – 4
Unacceptable – 0

Anchor statements outlining the expected general standard for each station are provided to all examiners in order to aid them reach their overall judgements.

A similar scale of marks will be awarded for the Clinical Video Scenarios Station. There will be a total of ten judgements.

A minimum score of 100 out of a maximum of 120 must be achieved to pass the examination.

Item analysis is undertaken on all theory examinations, providing statistics on overall test performance and individual test questions. This allows identification of any poorly discriminating items; all such questions are reviewed by the Angoff panels in advance of examination results being released and by the theory exam review group post-exam. This group scrutinises the item analysis data and makes edits to questions as appropriate.

Statistical reviews of the scenarios used as part of both the MRCPCH Clinical and DCH examinations are also undertaken, providing analysis of their overall performance and discriminative ability. This data is reviewed by the Communications and DCH board clinicians, and scenarios are edited as required to optimise their performance.

Quality assurance of RCPCH examiners both in the UK and Overseas continues to improve with the use of PERFORCE, which is an assessment of examiners discriminatory indices.

Since June 2007, the RCPCH has been providing examiners with feedback on their performance with regard to the MRCPCH Clinical exam; this feedback was also introduced for the DCH Clinical exam in 2013. Including a range of data, this analysis is sent in letter format to examiners after each clinical examination diet, providing them with some statistical data enabling them to review and calibrate their scoring over time. Examiners are provided with means and standard deviations of the marks they awarded, along with comparison data of other examiners: data on whether they are marking stringently or leniently (displayed as a 'Hawk-Dove Index' (HDI)) and data indicating whether they are able to rank candidates' performance and discriminate between well and poorly performing candidates. This data is received favourably by examiners.

The Psychometric Team also work on the development of new evaluation methods and ongoing enhancements of the current examinations. These provide opportunities to contribute to and undertake scientific research in the medical education field, which is presented at national and international conferences.

There are currently discussions with our European colleagues for the introduction of a common European paediatric examination.

The College works closely with the other Medical Royal College examination departments through the Academy of Medical Royal Colleges.

There are currently 450 UK examiners and 170 overseas covering nine MRCPCH clinical centres.

In the UK since 1999, 33,000 candidates have sat the written parts of the MRCPCH /DCH exam and since 2004, 13,800 the clinical examination.

Overseas, since 1999, 28,000 have taken the written examination, and since 2004, 4800 have taken the clinical exam.

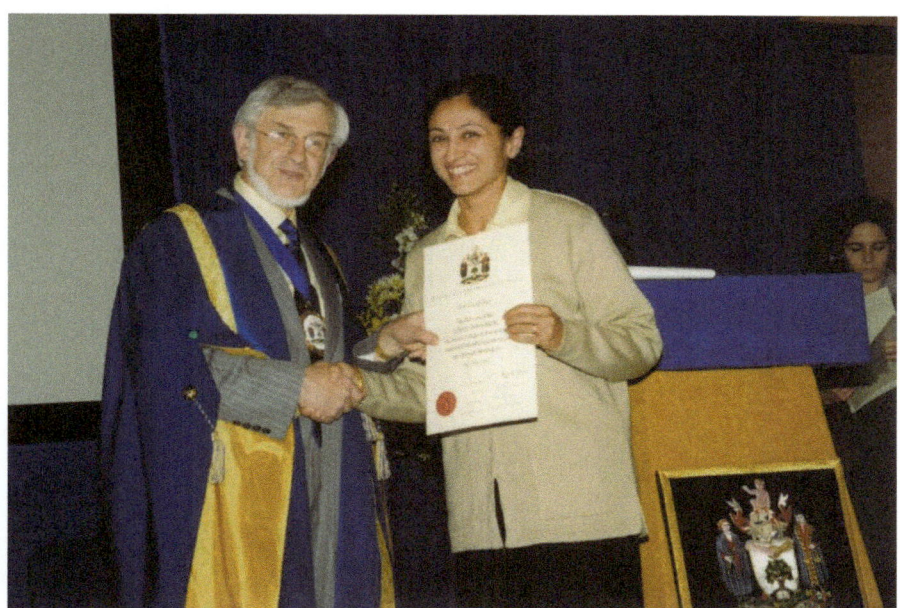

Presentation of MRCPCH diploma by Prof Sir David Hall

Training

10

Mary McGraw and Amanda Goldstein

Mary McGraw, a paediatric nephrologist in Bristol, oversaw the adoption by the College of its new responsibility for postgraduate training. Patricia Hamilton and Simon Newell also had enormous input into the development of our training programme. Amanda Goldstein is the current College Officer responsible for training.

Transition occurred at a time of great upheaval in training nationally, with the introduction of structured training programmes, making the task far more difficult.

Paediatric Training 1988–2014

Over the last two decades, there have been enormous changes in the training of paediatricians, and the role of the British Paediatric Association (BPA), and then the Royal College of Paediatrics and Child Health (RCPCH), in that training. Prior to the formation of the RCPCH, the responsibility for both trainees and training programmes were within the remit of the Royal Colleges of Physicians (RCP), although the BPA was very active in setting the standards. However, with the formation of the RCPCH all the responsibilities transferred to the College. There were also two major national initiatives, the Calman reforms and Modernising Medical Careers, that transformed the structure and delivery of training in all specialities which resulted in three distinct phases over this time: pre-Calman, post Calman and post Modernising Medical Careers.

M. McGraw (✉)
Bristol, UK

A. Goldstein
Birmingham, UK

© Springer International Publishing Switzerland 2017
A. Craft, K. Dodd (eds.), *From an Association to a Royal College*,
DOI 10.1007/978-3-319-43582-4_10

Pre-Calman

Prior to the Calman report (Sir Kenneth Calman was the chief medical officer for England) in 1993, training was delivered in three phases; senior house officer, registrar and senior registrar. The BPA was very active in setting standards not only for those training to be paediatricians but also worked closely with the Royal College of General Practitioners in setting standards for those who wished to become GPs. It was from this joint work on Child Health Surveillance that the first edition of Health for all Children was born. Although there was guidance on what constituted a training programme in the 'Blue Book', a publication of the Joint Committee on Higher Medical training of the RCP, doctors did not need to have completed that training programme in order to become a consultant. Visits to inspect training programmes were conducted by the Royal College of Physicians with the paediatric regional advisor providing the paediatric expertise.

It was the implications of the Calman reforms and the impact on training that was one of the strongest driving forces towards the formation of the RCPCH, in order to enable paediatricians to take full charge of the structure, standards and delivery of training.

The Calman report proposed that the duration and content of training should be clearly defined that Royal Colleges should specify the curriculum and that postgraduate deans should ensure the curriculum is delivered. It envisaged a shorter, more clearly defined period of training with the introduction of a combined training grade to replace registrars and senior registrars at the completion of which a Certificate of Completion of Specialist Training (CCST) would be awarded. The recommendations were accepted in December 1993. In response to this, the BPA produced 'Training in Paediatrics: Guidelines for Training Programmes' in 1994 and formed a committee, the Joint Committee of Higher Paediatric training (JCHPT), to discuss and design the processes which would need to underpin the training reforms. There was an emphasis on offering rotational training in both SHO and registrar posts to provide better continuity and avoiding the insecurity of frequent job hunting. Professor David Davies and Dr David Thistlethwaite led the development of a detailed syllabus for both basic specialist training and higher specialist training together with an SHO logbook. The transition process in the development of these reforms was a very busy time as at a local level regional advisors and College tutors not only had to restructure their training programmes, they also had to interview all those currently in registrar posts to see if they met the criteria to be assimilated into the new grade.

Post Calman

Implementation of the Calman report occurred in 1996, at the same time as the formation of the RCPCH, and saw the loss of the registrar and senior registrar grades with the formation of the new unified specialist registrar (SpR) grade in all specialties. The 'Orange guide' became the bible to which all those advising on training referred to guide trainees through the new regulations that governed this new training grade.

Five-year higher specialist training programmes in paediatrics were established that consisted of 2 years core training of neonates, community and general paediatrics followed by specialist training. This was the first time that any training in community paediatrics had become compulsory. At a local level, programme directors were appointed to run these programmes, and the role of the regional advisor greatly increased as they became the local leads for training on behalf of the RCPCH. With formation of a College, the RCPCH took full responsibility for training including quality assurance of training programmes and signing off CCSTs. A visit committee and two training committees replaced JCHPT to oversee these functions. A Paediatric Training Handbook (the 'Red Book') provided guidance on the structure of both basic specialist training (BST) and higher specialist training (HST). Introduction of the new regulations presented difficulties for some of those who had been training, often for many years and often by unorthodox routes, who found that they no longer met the criteria to enable them to complete training. College officers and College staff worked hard to deal with hundreds of distressed letters from bewildered doctors whilst trying to establish a record system that could cope. Taking on the roles and responsibilities for training at this time was a real baptism of fire!

In paediatrics there was a major expansion in specialist registrars who now had national training numbers (NTNs), the quantity of which was nationally decided. With the introduction of the NTN came the inevitable link between workforce planning and training and attempts to control the numbers entering training according to the predicted long-term service need. At this stage there was the concept that registrar numbers would be expanded temporarily in order to expand the numbers of consultants after which it would need to decrease. However the difficulties in predicting service needs together with factors influencing the length of training of individual doctors such as feminisation of the workforce and less than full-time training have continued to make workforce planning extremely difficult and still remains uncertain today.

A change in the visa regulations for workers coming from non-EU countries made a huge difference in the way doctors in training were recruited and left considerable gaps that were once filled by overseas doctors. Only designated shortage specialties were allowed to bypass the Tier 2 visa regulations, and for reasons that were not apparent, paediatrics in England and Wales was not designated as a shortage specialty. This was not the case in Scotland, so recruitment in Scotland followed the traditional pattern of the highest-scoring applicants who were appointed in order of merit. Elsewhere doctors from outside the UK/EU could only be appointed if UK/EU doctors did not meet the minimum requirements.

Led by Dr Janet Anderson as the Donald Court Fellow, a detailed and systematic programme of visiting took place. Units providing training were inspected against the standards set, and recommendations for improvement, where needed, were made together with planned systems put in place to ensure those recommendations were carried out. This had a significant impact on the quality of training and enabled the RCPCH to build up a detailed database on national training facilities. It became apparent through this process of visiting that although there was the ability to deliver standardised training in general paediatrics, there was a very variable access to tertiary specialty training throughout the country. This led to the birth of the 'National Grid' in 2003, an idea of Professor Sir Alan Craft, a process for ensuring equity of access to subspecialty training through a national appointment system. This also facilitated better matching of training numbers to consultant opportunities.

A system of College Specialist Advisory Committees (CSAC) was formed which allowed each of the subspecialties and eventually general paediatrics to have a significant input into the design of training programmes. They also became responsible for the assessment of progress of trainees and then for the recruitment to the National Grid training posts.

Modernising Medical Careers

Modernising Medical Careers led on from the Calman reforms 'to improve patient care by delivering a modernised and focussed career structure for doctors through a major reform in postgraduate education'. Starting with 'Unfinished Business' in 2002 proposing reforms of the SHO grade with a move towards programme-based training, the details were finalised in 'Modernising Medical Careers the next Steps' in 2004. In response to this, the RCPCH produced 'Training Paediatricians of the Future' which outlined the specialty training programme we have now of entering a run-through training grade with three levels of training, each supported by its own competency framework. Entry into Foundation programmes began in August 2005 with the first entry into specialty training in 2007. The 'Gold guide' became the new bible outlining the regulations.

The philosophy upon which the paediatric training programme was based was that becoming a consultant is dependent on competence, confidence and choice. The content, but not the length, of training programmes would be matched to suit a trainee's career path and the length of training could vary between 5 and 8 years dependant on the rate of progression of the trainee.

Competency frameworks were published for general paediatric training and all the subspecialties. During this time there was also a growth in the number of subspecialties with the recognition of four new subspecialties neurodisability, paediatric clinical pharmacology, paediatric intensive care and emergency medicine which then increased to 17, with the recognition of inherited metabolic disease and palliative care. In the cases of emergency medicine and paediatric intensive care, this involved close partnership working with other Colleges to develop joint programmes that could be entered from more than one specialty.

Linked to the competence frameworks was a detailed assessment strategy which introduced a range of workplace assessments to assess those competences. This became supported by the development of an eportfolio in 2007. All the workplace assessments were initially delivered via an external agent, but the RCPCH took over this process in 2010 with the development of its own assessment platform asset.

The medical royal colleges do not themselves have statutory responsibility for training, and all college curricula and assessment programmes need to go through rigorous approval processes by a statutory authority. The formation of the Postgraduate Medical Education and Training Board (PMETB) in 2005 amalgamated the roles of the two previous statutory authorities with responsibility for training: the Specialist Training Authority (STA) for hospital doctors and the Joint Committee on Training for General Practitioners (JCTGP) for GPs. It became responsible for all recommendations for the approval of training of both posts and individuals. PMETB took over the responsibility for quality assurance of training programmes and organised its own visits, and from this time visiting by the RCPCH ceased. It also took over the responsibility for assessing the training of those who had not followed conventional routes including those from overseas governed by the Article 14 of the General and Specialist Medical Practice (Education, Training and Qualifications) Order 2003. This is now known as the CESR route. Their decisions on paediatricians are based on recommendations made by the RCPCH. Establishing processes for approving all forms of training and making recommendations to PMETB demanded a huge input from College members and an increase in the numbers of College staff. All these roles have now transferred to the General Medical Council (GMC) after the merger of PMETB with the GMC in April 2010.

The Modernising Medical Careers initiative fell into disrepute by association with the recruitment scheme into training, the Medical Training Application Scheme (MTAS), which received a great deal of criticism and so was soon abandoned. However the RCPCH in 2008, based on its experience in national recruitment for tertiary training, was the first speciality to take on responsibility for recruitment into a subspecialty-specific standardised national process which was locally delivered. This has been highly successful and has become an established process which other colleges have now adopted.

Review of Modernising Medical Careers by Sir John Tooke suggested abandonment of run-through training, whereas the Department of Health response to that report recommended a mixed economy, with specialties choosing whether to retain a run-through programme or an uncoupled programme. The RCPCH chose to continue with a run-through programme which facilitates continuity by the delivery of a curriculum building on competences already gained and was favoured by trainees for allowing a better life work balance without the disruption of frequent geographical moves and career uncertainty. The College was fortunate that Dr Mary McGraw, strongly supported by Dr Patricia Hamilton, was taking a leading role in education and training at this crucial stage. The RCPCH is indebted to her for putting in place a training structure that is widely admired and has been a major factor in the success of achieving full recruitment of young doctors to our speciality.

Today the RCPCH continues to lead on a number of training reforms and has worked with other Colleges to develop a more broad-based training programme for those who are perhaps uncertain of their future career aims, and which could be entered from a number of specialties. Sadly Health Education England has suspended this successful programme. It was deemed too costly and took too long to get doctors particularly GPs into practice. Evidence from a Cardiff research group demonstrated that this was a very successful and popular programme with trainees learning holistic skills and decision-making.

Education Resources

The RCPCH wished to develop resources to facilitate local delivery of training and over the years has produced a number of successful e-learning packages to do this, in addition to running face-to-face courses including the Paediatric Educators' Programme to support those undertaking educational roles. Mastercourse, which underpins the whole of the level 1 curriculum and helps trainees prepare for the MRCPCH examination, was first conceived in 2000. The original project failed as the publishers realised that the final product would cost too much to produce. However thanks to the persistence of Professor Malcolm Levene, who remained enthusiastic about the project, alternative publishers were sought, and a two-volume written learning package, together with a DVD of clinical material, began development in 2002 and was finally published in 2007. It has proved a very popular resource for those preparing for examinations both in the UK and abroad. Collaboration with other groups with expertise in developing e-learning programmes such as the Advanced Life Support Group (ALSG) and e-Learning for Health (e-lfH) has resulted in further educational resources on safeguarding children and young people and the adolescent health programme, all of which can be used by those in training as well as for continuing professional development of trained doctors. Continuing provision of resources to support training and professional development remains a priority for the College for the future.

There have been huge changes in training and education over the last two decades; the BPA and the RCPCH are proud to have been proactive in responding to those changes, often leading developments that are then adopted by other colleges. However we cannot be complacent as this is an area in which continuing change will occur, and with it the need to remain ready to continue to grow and develop.

Not only health care but also education provision was affected by the 2012 Health and Social Care Act, which led to the fragmentation of providers of doctors' education. Health Education England took on oversight and leadership for professional education and training with deaneries being replaced by Local Education and Training Boards (LETB); LETBs had responsibility for all health-care staff training. This caused concern within the medical fraternity that the expensive and lengthy medical postgraduate paediatric training would be disadvantaged. In addition Public Health England emerged, and an attempt to allow paediatricians' access to child public health training has become more difficult.

These education boards (previously deaneries) have responsibility for annual assessment of trainees and determining their appropriate progress (Annual Review of Competency Progression – ARCP). In the past this may have been done by face-to-face contact with the trainees, but now LETBs undertake the ARCP electronically from a distance though may arrange annual face-to-face career planning meetings. Trainees who are not progressing satisfactorily may have to have targeted training or even be released from training. The processes for this have become more robust with specific guidance available through the Gold Guide, the Reference Guide to Postgraduate Speciality Training (produced and revised regularly by the Conference of Postgraduate Medical Deans). With tighter supervision and assessment, the increasing tendency of trainees to appeal against decisions made against them has come. Better organisation of paediatric subspecialty training through the National Grid process led to the need for CSACs to monitor their trainees more closely. They are now expected to assess their trainees' progress annually and feed this into the ARCP process. This is considerable extra work for large CSACs such as neonatal and Community Child Health and the need for a lead for these subspecialties in every region evolved. In 2015, the Community Child Health training programme became the most recent programme to become part of the National Grid process.

It also became clear that there was a need for an assessment for paediatricians coming to the end of their training, and hence START (Specialty Training Assessment of Readiness for Tenure) was born. This was initially known as ST7 assessment and is a formative assessment for trainees in level 3 training and most taking it in ST7. The format is OSCE based, and scenarios reflect the dilemmas faced by consultants on a regular basis such as prioritising on a ward round, dealing with prescription errors and communication with colleagues.

Assessment methods have changed dramatically in the last 5 years. The most recent format has given the clinical supervisors the option of white space for comment only and not using a numerical scoring system. A consequence has been that many of the assessments are more formative and are certainly more useful to the trainee. New types of assessments have evolved, and trainees now have to demonstrate their competence in leadership, acute care of the seriously ill child, as well as written communication, and handover. These 'supervised learning events' are amongst the many workplace-based assessments required of a trainee throughout their training.

Recording of trainees' achievements and progress has become fully electronic, and the eportfolio is the way of things! For the first time in a decade, the college has made a full and comprehensive overhaul of the system used, and the new eportfolio became live in early 2016. It has been one of the most difficult changes as all existing data in the old system had to be completely transferred with no omissions. As the ARCP is electronic, the importance of getting this right could not be overemphasised.

Electronic systems have also made it possible to complete all the written exams on computer rather than paper, and from 2015 candidates could take any of these papers throughout the UK in designated exam centres (many regions used driving test centres) both in the UK and overseas. The result of this is that trainees do not have so far to travel, the supervision of the exam can be done by trained centre staff and the results available sooner. Other changes to the exam system mean that trainees can take the three written papers (Theory and Science, Foundation of Practice, Applied Knowledge in Practice) in any order.

Many trainees are now applying to take time out of their training programme to experience work overseas and undertake research programmes. Some of this is humanitarian work, and there has been an expansion of the facility for trainees to work with organisations such as VSO or college sponsored links to resource-poor countries. This is popular amongst trainees, many of whom have expressed interest in global child health. Although not an option for all subspecialty trainees, some CSACs encourage work in countries with well-developed health systems, and some paediatric intensive care trainees spend a year in Canada or Australia. In addition, the RCPCH has developed links with resource-poor countries to offer training in the UK. This is known as the Medical Training Initiative and offers 2 years of UK paediatric training for senior trainees from West Africa and other regions.

As well as the option for subspecialty training, there has been the evolution of special interest modules (SPIN) for general paediatricians in the third stage of training. These programmes are now more structured with designated supervisors, assessment methods and CSAC sign off. Some are very popular particularly epilepsy and diabetes, and the RCPCH is piloting the completion of SPIN modules by consultants. Although most SPIN modules have originated in and are monitored by the RCPCH, there are some, e.g. paediatric dermatology and paediatric cardiology, that require close relationship with the Royal College of Physicians. Some topics are not suitable for SPIN module development but are very good training opportunities which trainees can take out of programme to pursue paediatric public health, global child health and paediatric audiology. It is possible that in the future, these SPIN modules may evolve into credentials as has been proposed as part of the Shape of Training recommendations.

The Shape of Training report from Professor David Greenaway in 2013 had a profound effect on the way training has been viewed both through the RCPCH and other medical royal colleges. Its proposals questioned the length of training and the relevance of training programmes for modern health-care needs given problems of the elderly, frail and multiply morbid patient whilst maintaining general and acute care skills. It suggested that there would be lifelong learning through 'credentialing' and ability for trainees to move between specialties through a system of shared competencies. Breaking down the primary/secondary care boundaries and increased 'generalism' is a key recommendation of this report. This has implications for the future though we have not seen any of the proposals implemented yet. The RCPCH has determined to keep any review of its curriculum 'shape compliant' but has resisted attempt to shorten training. The plan is to continue with the flexible approach of our three-tiered programme with the ability to shorten each stage if competencies are achieved sooner. There is an understandable and laudable wish to see enhanced training in the paediatrics that is practiced outside of hospitals and in primary care and the converse that every GP should have appropriate training in the care of children.

The General Medical Council (GMC) having taken over the responsibility for medical students, doctors in training and doctors not in training has been much more prescriptive about the expectation of how the profession should practice. Their Good Medical Practice, updated in 2013, outlines these expectations and responsibilities of doctors. They are also developing general professional capabilities, which will guide the educational outcomes expected of doctors in training. All curricula will need to show how doctors can meet these expectations. The RCPCH is in the process of having the first major curriculum review for 10 years, and this is timely given the GMC expectations. It comes at the time of the eportfolio revision, and it is anticipated that the new curriculum will be fully electronic and allow trainees to record and monitor their training more easily.

Of course it would be impossible to write about training without reference to the inevitable tension between service and training. The RCPCH documents Facing the Future (2011 and revised 2015) recognises that it would be impossible to meet the standards recommended with the current workforce whilst allowing trainees to access educational opportunities. By suggesting innovative ways of working, for example, different consultant shifts, paediatric assessment units and the appropriate training and employment of specialist nurses and physician associates, it has hoped to redress this balance. The European Working Time Directive protected current paediatricians in training from the arduous and potentially harmful shifts of the previous generations but has changed the structure of daytime working with less time for undertaking clinics and less direct supervision by a consultant mentor. The Temple Report (Time for Training 2010) recognised this and was at pains to point out the need to make every training opportunity count, noting that working alongside a consultant in an evening shift would have considerable educational value for a trainee. This report also highlighted the great importance and value of training and trainers to the NHS. The widely quoted 'better training better care' was one of the first times high-quality training was specifically acknowledged to contribute to better health-care outcomes.

The RCPCH has recognised its role in the training not only of paediatricians but all those who work with children. There have been increasing numbers of paediatric and neonatal nurse practitioners, some now are using the eportfolio as a pilot. We are working together with the RCGP to assist in improving the training offered to GPs. The importance of this was stressed by Sir Ian Kennedy in 2010 who recognised that children's health in the UK lagged behind Europe and attributed this in part to the lack of knowledge of children's illness by GPs. Physician associates are now working in paediatric units, and although the RCPCH does not have direct responsibility for their training, paediatricians do contribute to their training.

Further Reading

1. Department of Health. Hospital doctors: training for the future. The report of the working group on specialist medical training. London: DoH; 1993.
2. Hall D. Health for all Children. 1st ed. Oxford University Press, 1989.
3. Department of health A Guide to Specialist Registrar training March 2006.
4. Royal College of Paediatrics and Child Health Paediatric Training Handbook. 1st ed. London: RCPCH; 2003.
5. Royal College of Paediatrics and Child Health Paediatric Training Handbook. 2nd ed. London: RCPCH; 2008.
6. McGraw M, Ng G. The Royal College of Paediatrics and Child health programme for subspecialty training. Arch Dis Child. 2006;91:71–3.
7. Department of health Sir Liam Donaldson Unfinished Business: proposals for the SHO grade August 2002
8. Department of health Modernising Medical Careers The next steps: the future shape of Foundation, Specialist and General Practice Training Programmes April 2004
9. Royal College of Training Paediatrics and Child Health Training Paediatricians of the future June 2004.
10. Royal College of Paediatrics and Child Health Training Paediatricians of the future 2005 update.
11. Royal College of Paediatrics and Child Health A Framework of competences for Basic Specialist Training October 2004.
12. Royal College of Paediatrics and Child Health A Framework of competences for Core Higher Specialist Training in Paediatrics October 2005.
13. Royal College of Paediatrics and Child Health A Framework of Competences for level 3 Training July 2006.
14. UK Departments of Health. A Guide to Postgraduate Medical training. 1st ed. 2007.
15. Sir John Tooke Aspiring to Excellence; Final Report of the Independent Inquiry into Modernising Tooke Report November 2008 Medical Careers January 2008.
16. Department of Health Implementing the Health and Social Care Act 2012 Department of Health http://www.dh.gov.uk/healthandsocialcarebill.
17. Shape of Training report 2013 Professor Greenaway http://www.shapeoftraining.co.uk/static/documents/content/Shape_of_training_FINAL_Report.pdf_53977887.pdf.
18. GMC Good Medical Practice 2013. http://www.gmc-uk.org/guidance/good_medical_practice.asp.
19. Facing the Future RCPCH revised 2015. http://www.rcpch.ac.uk/facingthefuture.
20. Temple Report – Time for Training 2010.
21. Getting it right for Children and Young People Professor Sir Ian Kennedy 2010.

Growth of Specialties and Specialist Societies

11

Roy Meadow

Roy Meadow here reflects on the growth of the paediatric subspecialties. The two largest are those for perinatal medicine and community child health and we have asked Peter Dunn and Simon Lenton to give some more detail. A full list of current specialty groups and special interest groups can be found on the RCPCH website.

This account considers specialties within paediatrics itself, and not those other important paediatric specialties within surgery, psychiatry and other disciplines. The current comprehensive range of specialty services for children throughout the UK has grown on the template set 40 years ago.

In many ways the development of paediatric subspecialists echoes that of Britain's first paediatricians. The early days were reliant on adult specialty physicians and then came general paediatricians who had a special interest in particular disorders, before there were part-time paediatric specialists whose major work was still general paediatrics. Now trainees can select a specialty early in their career, receive formal training in that specialty and become full-time paediatric specialists.

That gradual evolution was inevitable. More than 20 years after the inauguration of the NHS, many large cities and several counties in Britain continued to have a single or at the most two paediatricians; they had to be generalists. Even by 1970 when I went to Leeds as a paediatric senior lecturer, I became one of only five consultant paediatricians serving a population of over 800,000, with child inpatients in 11 different hospitals, newborns in 4 different hospitals, 2 of which were more than 30 miles apart, as well as considerable community and regional responsibilities. Rationalising those services and creating facilities suitable for children and their parents were the priorities, and more important than developing paediatric specialties. At that time, whatever a paediatrician's special interest, their primary

R. Meadow
Leeds, Uk

© Springer International Publishing Switzerland 2017
A. Craft, K. Dodd (eds.), *From an Association to a Royal College*,
DOI 10.1007/978-3-319-43582-4_11

responsibility had to be as a generalist. Even Great Ormond Street Hospital, unencumbered by the need to provide a local, community or neonatal service, only had two or three specialist paediatricians for much of the 1970s; most were generalists with a special interest. In later years the hospital became an important centre for specialist services and training.

The small number of paediatricians in the UK was a big reason why the development of subspecialities was more than 10 years behind that in adult medicine and many decades behind that in North America. Nevertheless the 1970s saw the start of changes, which were influenced by several factors including:

Paediatric Cardiology

Paediatric cardiology was one of the first specialties to develop, and in most regions owed its development to the ingenuity and hard work of adult cardiologists who adapted their skills to provide a service for neonates and children. The resulting regional centres for paediatric cardiology provided a very good service, but one with particular problems for paediatricians. Often infants and young children were cared for in isolated regional adult units, converted from old TB sanatoria, where there were no children-trained staff, inadequate facilities for children and families and laboratories that required 5–10 ml of blood in order to measure electrolyte levels. It was difficult for paediatricians to influence arrangements at an adult unit where they did not work, and meetings with the adult cardiologists were not easy: the main allegiances of those pioneering paediatric cardiologists were to the Colleges of Physicians and the British Cardiac Society, not to the BPA. The BPA was concerned that cardiology could set the pattern for other paediatric specialties and that organ/system specialty care of children could become the domain of adult specialists.

Paediatric Training

Training had become better organised, more formal, but also more rigid. It was usual for the trainee to work for 2 years as a middle-grade registrar, followed by 4 years as a senior registrar, half of that time being in hospitals outside the university regional centre. Whether in or out of the centre, the jobs had heavy service commitments on which the host unit relied. Excellent general experience was gained, without the chance to develop a major special interest. More flexible training programmes were possible for university staff. Outside London, large university departments of Paediatrics and Child Health had developed led by professors, with freedom from central university targets or research assessment exercises, who saw their role as developing comprehensive services for children in their region, including the creation of paediatric specialties. Notable exceptions to that pattern were two London departments at The Hammersmith and at University College where Professors Tizard and Strang concentrated resources on perinatology, research and the training of academic leaders. Elsewhere, members of university departments were encouraged to have different specialist interests. For instance, in a unit of one professor, two senior lecturers (honorary consultants) and four lecturers/tutors (honorary registrars), one would concentrate on neonatology and others on gastroenterology, nephrology, endocrinology, neurology, etc. The junior university grade staff had personalised training programmes allowing them to achieve specialty training in the USA and Canada or in adult specialty units in the UK. Very soon, regardless of relatively junior appointments, they were running specialist units in their teaching hospital which became regional paediatric referral units. There were examples of regional services for oncology, receiving 70 new cases a year, being run by a lecturer of registrar status. Well into the 1980s, most of those leading paediatric specialty services and their regional referral units were university staff.

Clinical Responsibility

Whether employed by the NHS or the university, trainees of that time had great clinical responsibility and also freedom to innovate. They were responsible to a general paediatrician who knew little of the subspecialty that their registrar was learning from colleagues who were abroad, in adult departments or similarly placed in other paediatric departments. They got on with the job, unhampered by conservative advice from senior consultants. The first successful haemodialysis of a young child with acute renal failure was done by a paediatric senior registrar working with the preregistration house officer and the senior house officer in adult medicine; the paediatrician nominally in charge, an expert in neuro-development, was told about it several days afterwards.

European and British Specialist Societies

Contact between those developing a specialty was crucial at a time when senior colleagues were mainly generalists. The European paediatric specialist societies were important places for learning, sharing ideas, improving training and for collaborative clinical research, particularly before a country had sufficient numbers in a specialty to warrant a national society. In nephrology, for example, it was not until 8 specialists from the UK and Ireland were attending European Paediatric Nephrology meetings that the 8 decided to form a British Association for Paediatric Nephrology, which at its first meeting in 1973 had 15 members.

In those times both the BPA and the university professors recognised that specialties should develop and hoped that it could occur within paediatrics rather than from adult specialties; there was uncertainty about the process. There were specific concerns about organisation and responsibility for training, and fears that paediatric organ specialists could drift away to adult organ societies, losing ties to paediatrics in general, and the BPA in particular. This was a great fear for those who wanted a College.

BPA Annual Meetings

For several decades the pattern of the Annual meeting had been a series of plenary sessions mostly of mixed content. At the 1971 meeting in Lancaster, there was an important innovation which had big consequences. For the first time, there was an afternoon in which there were two concurrent sessions, one of which was devoted to endocrinology. The background was that limited supplies of growth hormone (GH), from cadaver pituitary, had become available to approved units with facilities to measure accurately both GH and children. (The unforeseen tragedy was that those deemed safe to issue GH perforce became licensed distributors of Jakob-Creutzfeldt disease.) This group of paediatricians with a special interest in endocrinology met regularly and called themselves the British Paediatric Endocrinology Group (BPEG).

The academic board thought it likely that BPEG would request a session at future annual meetings and realised that the group model could be the way forwards for the development of paediatric specialties, ensuring support from, and representation within, the BPA and a good way to develop the annual meeting and ensure its attraction for subspecialists. There followed a time of great activity by the academic board to persuade paediatricians with a special interest to form specialty groups within, or linked to, the BPA.

The BPA's enticements included sessions at the annual meeting, representation on training and other relevant committees and financial or secretarial help. The response from the specialists was usually positive, but a recurrent fear was of too much control by the BPA or damage to the important membership most of the specialists had in societies such as The British Society for Gastroenterology or The Renal Association. Neonatologists were among the most resistant because their leaders belonged to the prestigious multidisciplinary Neonatal Society and did not want another association or potential interference from the BPA, (who wanted groups to be open to any member with a special interest and not confined to a self-selected clique). It was not until several years later that Peter Dunn was able to persuade and lead his colleagues to form the British Association for Perinatal Medicine. The development of groups led to a long-lasting change in the form of the BPA annual meeting and its venues. Traditionally there had been 2–3 days of plenary sessions, but by 1975 the number of concurrent group sessions demanded a university campus, York, with plentiful lecture rooms. By 2000, ten or more concurrent group session took place on most afternoons.

The Autonomy of Groups

This was always contentious, and its extent varied between groups. Realistically the BPA had to allow considerable autonomy at first in order to attract and retain its system specialists. It has also had some unforeseen benefits: there have been many times in the last 30 years when a BPA/College president has been more pleased than irritated by a specialty group going direct to the minister or the media, fighting their corner on behalf of their patients, with a single-mindedness that would be inappropriate for a president representing many different interests.

From the beginning of specialisation, the concerns were greatest for those with major links to adult organ specialties. None doubted that specialists dealing with neonates or disabled, disadvantaged or abused children would retain their strongest links with the BPA/RCPCH, but there were realistic concerns that the organ/system specialists would see their home as the adult specialist societies and their colleges. Now they form a major part of the membership of our College. The paediatric organ specialists have used their autonomy wisely, and though working mainly through the RCPCH, have retained important links with the corresponding adult society. Most have their main scientific meeting at the College annual meeting in the spring and a major independent meeting later in the year sometimes with an adult society or another paediatric specialist group.

The British Association of Perinatal Medicine (BAPM)

12

Peter Dunn

Peter Dunn who worked in Bristol was one of the pioneers of neonatal paediatrics. He was instrumental in establishing BAPM and here gives a brief overview.

At the end of the 1980s as the British Paediatric Association was working to emerge as a separate entity outside the umbrella of the Royal College of Physicians, the British Association of Perinatal Medicine was continuing the work of trying to establish specialist perinatal care. Throughout that decade the differentiation of obstetric units and neonatal units into those offering complex care and those that offered a less specialist service to a local population had made little progress or indeed no progress in some parts of the UK. At that stage neither the BPA nor the Royal College of Obstetrics and Gynaecology (RCOG) fully recognised the need to establish a coordinated specialist neonatology and high-risk obstetric service across the country. However it was at the end of the 1980s, as therapeutic options began to grow, that there was a growing recognition of a role for specialist neonatology and neonatal centres, even though the vast majority of specialist neonatal care was delivered by consultants who had both paediatric and neonatal patients and who worked outside the specialist neonatal centres. It is probably fair to say it was large outside influences which drove a major change in this situation.

The first change in the early 1990s was therapeutic. The trials and subsequent licensing of surfactant for the use in respiratory distress syndrome led to dramatic improvements in survival. Almost simultaneously the potential benefit of antenatal steroids in improving outcomes for preterm babies was recognised. As a consequence neonatal medicine was able to realistically offer treatment to a wider group of babies and with the expectation of good outcomes. As a result attitudes to the

P. Dunn
Bristol, UK

© Springer International Publishing Switzerland 2017
A. Craft, K. Dodd (eds.), *From an Association to a Royal College*,
DOI 10.1007/978-3-319-43582-4_12

provision of specialist neonatal intensive care became increasingly positive in association with rising expectations amongst staff and the general public.

The second change was organisational. Although the 'purchaser/provider split' of the very early 1990s had a negative effect on the formation of specialist neonatology in that it encouraged units of all types to provide the full range of neonatal care for their own babies, it did, for the first time in the UK, highlight the issue of the cost of service provision. This had never really been seriously considered in the UK and led to a realisation that neonatal intensive care was potentially expensive and should be organised in the most cost-effective manner possible. In the mid 1990s, the Calman reforms of medical training had a far bigger influence in starting a process that culminated some years later in the development of the various specialist roles within paediatrics, and one of these was neonatology. The Calman reforms introduced both regulation of the hours that junior doctors could work and placed greater emphasis, for the first time, on the training role of these posts. As a consequence the task of supervision and quality assurance of training became an issue.

When the Royal College of Paediatrics and Child Health was formed, it took some time for the nature of the relationship with BAPM to emerge, i.e. who did what? The College invited BAPM to have a major role in the specialist committee overseeing neonatal training, and similarly RCPCH met regularly with all of the various subspecialty groups including BAPM. The training role remains and although the relevant committee is a College subcommittee, it is led by BAPM. Regular meetings between the College and the various subspecialty interest groups and organisations ceased in the early years of the new century. Subsequently there has been good collaboration between BAPM and the College on a number of topics of joint interest, but there has been no forum where the two organisations regularly interact since that time. However issues of specialist neonatology were seen increasingly as the province of BAPM. In recent years requests for advice from official bodies have generally gone to both organisations, whereas in the 1990s, they went to the BPA/RCPCH and were sometimes, but not always, shared. This change is perhaps a sign that the two organisations have both now developed a more clear-cut identity

A similar process took place in relation to specialist obstetrics and the RCOG. Perhaps because the majority of the initial members of the fledgling BAPM were from a paediatric background, much of the business of the BAPM executive was 'neonatal'. This is despite an executive structure that was balanced between neonatologists and those with an obstetric background. Perhaps for this reason, at around the time the reforms to medical training began, a parallel organisation to BAPM, focussing on specialist obstetric care, was formed: the British Maternal and Fetal Medicine Society (BMFMS). The RCOG was much slower to recognise specialist obstetric care than RCPCH in relation to neonatology, but nonetheless the formation of BMFMS was the catalyst for the situation that now exists:

• Two Royal Colleges that cover their entire relevant specialist field
• Each with specialist societies that cover particular areas of specialist practice (although RCOG also has a formal recognition of BAPM as one of the specialist societies with which it liaises)

One consequence of this greater polarisation of the business of BAPM to neonatology has been its development as a multidisciplinary organisation with members from a wide range of backgrounds including management, nursing and dietetics. This change into an organisation with a clear focus on neonatal issues has influenced the relationship between BAPM and RCPCH. Increasingly it seems that the College sets a broad agenda (e.g. training, work force, revalidation), whilst specialty issues (neonatal standards, issues of specialist service delivery such as cooling) are the domain of BAPM.

Of course the organisational changes in the delivery of neonatal care following a Department of Health review in 2003 involving the formation of networks and the designation of units have been part of this process of increasing specialisation. Hours regulation and the network structure have led to the appointment of more specialist neonatologists, and many of these clinicians see themselves as 'not trained' to deal with older paediatric patients. In contrast paediatricians who work in district general hospitals are often involved in more basic neonatal care and sometimes short-term intensive care. These differences in role mirror the focus of the two organisations. The same appears true in relation to the scientific meetings run by RCPCH and BAPM (where the needs, as perceived by the members of the two organisations, are generally quite different).

This separation of roles has increased the possibility of fragmentation. At the time of writing whilst there is no formal relationship in terms of liaison with RCPCH, on the whole informal liaison continues to work well, but this has benefitted from the presence of many neonatologists or paediatricians with a strong interest in neonatal care amongst the College officers since its formation.

The British Association for Community Child Health (BACCH) Formerly the Community Paediatric Group (CPG)

13

Simon Lenton

Community paediatrics has developed over the last 40 years since the importance of the care of children outside of hospital was recognised. Donald Court in his review of Child Health Services recommended the development of consultant community paediatric posts. Simon Lenton, who is a consultant community paediatrician in Bath here describes the development of the specialist society, BACCH. He was a College Vice president for health services from 2004–2009.

Introduction

BACCH is the largest specialty group within the Royal College of Paediatrics and Child Health (RCPCH), and this chapter reviews the origins of BACCH and its influence both within the college and on the development of community child health services for families throughout the UK.

Central to the development of community child health services has been the development of leadership and clinical expertise through the appointment of consultant paediatricians in community child health (CPCCH) and then the development of subspecialties within community child health, such as disability, public health, audiology, child protection and child mental health, in order to meet the ever-changing morbidity in childhood.

BACCH continues to advocate for family-centred care provided in local communities, promoting health using a life course approach and service development based on pathways, delivered by networks which strive for continuous quality improvement in experience and outcomes. To achieve this BACCH works closely

S. Lenton
Bath, UK

© Springer International Publishing Switzerland 2017
A. Craft, K. Dodd (eds.), *From an Association to a Royal College*,
DOI 10.1007/978-3-319-43582-4_13

with other professional groups within health and other agencies and closely with the RCPCH.

History

The history of BACCH must be viewed simultaneously alongside the position of children in society and changes in childhood morbidity, the wider socio-political changes of the late twentieth century, particularly reorganisation of the National Health Service (NHS), with more community-based service provision coupled and newly available health interventions.

The roots of Community Child Health started with public health interventions of the late nineteenth century and with a medical and nursing workforce which expanded throughout the mid-twentieth century with a peak in the 1950s and 1960s. This workforce was employed by local authorities, often led by community medicine specialists, and it was not until the 1974 reorganisation that this workforce joined the NHS.

The history of BACCH is essentially the story of how the work of this community child health workforce evolved and became integrated into the NHS, and this chapter is presented in three decades.

1976–1985: The Beginnings

The publication in 1976 of "Fit for the Future", the report of the Committee on Child Health Services chaired by Donald Court, was the seminal point in the development of Community Child Health services as we know them today. The report acknowledged the health gains made by children over the previous century but looked to the future and recommended improved community-based, integrated care, led by paediatricians, particularly for children with long-term conditions.

The origins/initiation of the British Association for Community Child Health (BACCH) was recorded as a request from John Davies, then chair of the Academic Board of the British Paediatric Association requesting that the BPA "wanted to have contact with, and at times advice from, a group of community paediatricians. Such a group would be associated, but not part of the BPA". Frank Bamford took this forward during the BPA meeting in Harrogate in April 1974 when he met with a small group of like-minded paediatricians to propose the "British Association of Community Paediatrics" whose first formal meeting was on 23 October 1974. The stated purpose of the group was "to contribute to the improvement in the care of all children, to promote scientific study of clinical community paediatrics, to facilitate the exchange of knowledge, information and ideas among its members and to disseminate knowledge of clinical community paediatrics" (the word children includes adolescents).

However, the British Paediatric Association objected to the title of "British Association of Community Paediatrics", and after protracted discussions for over 2 years, the name was amended to the Community Paediatric Group and finally adopted on 11 November 1976. The group remained independent of the BPA until 1984 when the BPA formally recognised the CPG by setting up a BPA Liaison Group "to consider issues relating to community paediatrics".

During this first decade, the Community Paediatric Group spent considerable time defining the role and duties of a consultant paediatrician in community child health and lobbying the BPA to include community child health as a legitimate specialty within paediatrics. While the BPA paper "Paediatric manpower: towards the twenty-first century" in 1984 acknowledged roles of consultant community paediatricians, they also assumed these consultants would contribute to the acute hospital call rota, thus effectively transferring community resources into hospital settings.

The other problem revolved around the fact that the majority of doctors (CMOs and SCMOs) working in community settings with children often had no formal postgraduate qualifications other than experience and on-the-job training. The BPA as the "governing body" for the education and training of paediatricians did not feel these doctors were "paediatricians", and as the majority were not members of the BPA, they did not feel responsible for their education and training.

The CPG repeatedly described the role of a consultant paediatrician in community child health (CPCCH) in the early 1980s, but it was not until the Child Health Forum produced a report in 1988, linked to the BPA census, which identified 47 CPCCH (working more than five sessions a week in community child health) recommended one CPCCH per district and recognised that further expansion would be required in the future that the BPA acknowledged the need for workforce planning and formal training programmes for these consultants.

1985–1994: Development of Community Child Health

Having proved the need for CPCCH, the Joint Committee on Higher Medical Training (JCHMT) of the Royal College of Physicians (London) produced a model training programme which in 1985 enabled the development of senior registrar training posts. The mismatch between people in training and the numbers of senior doctors retiring from established community child health departments soon became apparent. The CPG responded by producing a number of workforce planning documents throughout this decade arguing for an expansion of both consultant numbers and training programmes.

One particular area of concern was of public health. After lobbying the BPA and Faculty of Community Medicine, a joint working party was formed to examine the interface between public health and child health. The outcome was a paper entitled "Working Together for Tomorrow's Children" in 1998 which helpfully defined the needs of local populations and the roles and responsibilities of each professional group.

In 1989 the publication of the first of the "Hall reports" (Health for All Children) covering preschool child health surveillance was seen. This was one of the earliest reports to apply evidence-based medicine approaches to clinical services to create a national framework for preschool surveillance. The initial report focused on the screening components within child health surveillance and acknowledged that the evidence base for many of surveillance and promotion activities was lacking. The result was that child health surveillance was cut back to the core of what was considered essential.

From the perspective of community child health services, this was the start of a major evolutionary process from a comprehensive public health-orientated, whole population service delivered by a combined workforce of largely clinical medical officers, health visitors and school nurses, to a secondary care community child health service focusing on long-term conditions and vulnerable families, delivered by consultant paediatricians, staff and associate grade specialists and increasingly trainees.

All the routine surveillance and health promotion would eventually transfer to primary care teams, and all the local authority specialist services are largely integrated into hospital-based care, for example, orthopaedics. The acceptance and endorsement of the role of consultant leadership within community child health services led to the transition of the Community Paediatric Group into the British Association for Community Child Health in 1992. The change of name (for child health) was a deliberate emphasis to focus on improving child health rather than representing the interests of paediatricians (of community paediatricians) or a focus on disease (of community paediatrics). The reasons for the change of name eventually influenced the name and focus of the BPA as it transitioned to later become the Royal College of Paediatrics and Child Health thanks to the influence of David Baum, who had been the chair of BACCH.

One of the first publications BACCH produced was a detailed syllabus of training, based on knowledge and skills, to guide the expansion and training of senior registrars in community child health.

BACCH also produced a number of workforce planning documents indicating the number of senior registrars required to replace retiring senior clinical medical officers (SCMOs). This initiated a prolonged regrading process of SCMOs (child health) into CPCCH posts.

The introduction of the NHS internal market with GP fundholders created considerable anxiety for those providing services not primarily driven by GP referrals. The response from BACCH was to produce a guide for purchasers and providers entitled "Services for Children" a model for purchasers and paediatricians in 1994 which laid down an approach based on pathways of care, provided by five teams covering acute and long-term illness, disability, social paediatrics, behavioural paediatrics and public health, a framework later adopted by the National Service Framework 15 years later.

As consultant leadership of these teams developed, the need for and roles of specialist expertise within community child health became apparent. The BPA was unwilling to recognise the specialist groups within community child health, and so it was agreed that BACCH would act as an umbrella organisation to represent these interests.

The development of specialty groups in some ways mirrors the development of BACCH starting with a few enthusiasts developing the specialty, recognition of that specialty and then the need for training and accreditation, followed by workforce planning and practical service delivery. The British Academy of Childhood Disability was the first to gain RCPCH specialty recognition.

The two-day Annual Scientific Meeting of BACCH allows specialty groups the opportunity to present both research and share best practice in their areas as the majority of CPCCH are generalists.

The BACCH response to the Calman training reforms in 1994 was to develop programmes where generic community child health training occurred over 2 years, with a third year within a chosen specialty.

Safeguarding became an increasingly important part of the role of CCH, and this is described in the chapter by Sibert and Debelle.

1995–2004: Embedding Community Child Health

This decade started with the publication of the Polnay Report, *Health needs of school age children* in 1995 which extended the preschool focus in Health for All Children up into the school age. The conclusions were that routine surveillance was outdated and the service should concentrate on those children with medical, social or psychological problems. The role of the school nurse was promoted and the role of the school doctor contracted and was no longer school-based.

The upheaval in provision of preschool and school health was followed in 1996 by the Department of Health publication "Child Health in the Community: A Guide to Good Practice" led by Jerry Reid in which for the first time the Department of Health attempted to establish uniformity of the provision of community child health services in the UK.

In 1996 the formation of the RCPCH was a milestone for the development of community-based services for children and families since child health was firmly included within the remit of the new college. The publications by the RCPCH in early 2002 of "The Next 10 years: Educating Paediatricians for New Roles in the 21st Century" and the report "Strengthening the Care of Children in the Community: A Review of Community Child Health" both acknowledged that the boundaries between hospital-based and community-based practice were becoming increasingly blurred and that training in community child health, particularly relating to the subspecialist areas notably disability, child protection and social paediatrics, child mental health and educational medicine and child public health required further attention and investment. Additionally, for the first time, there was discussion about the configuration of paediatrics and health services and the need for reconfiguration and a comprehensive workforce review covering community, hospital and specialist paediatric workforces.

2005–2014: Improving Community Child Health

This decade started with the publication of the Children and Young People's National Service Framework from the Department of Health (DH) and the Children Act from the Department of Education and Skills (DfES).

The Children and Young People's NSF had reinforced the need for integrated working in teams crossing primary, secondary and tertiary healthcare and between health, education, social care and the voluntary sector. Services planned, delivered and improved based on pathway approaches and delivered by teams working in partnership with families were recommended.

BACCH worked closely with the RCPCH in producing Modelling the Future which consisted of three linked publications between 2007 and 2009 outlining the need for the reconfiguration of services, reduction in the number of units providing inpatient care, development of more comprehensive community services and investment in quality improvement and learning especially in times of change.

The 2012 Health and Social Care Act replaced 152 primary care trusts with 211 GP-led clinical commissioning groups and a single NHS Commissioning Board for England. The impact was that many community child health services previously hosted by primary care trusts had to find new organisations to host their services. Some elected to merge with hospital services, and others formed social enterprise organisations, while others merged with existing community-based organisations.

The transfer of public health functions (in England) to local authorities and the loss of relationships with previous commissioners within PCTs have created considerable concern, as the focus of the new commissioners was largely on high-cost secondary care rather than balanced with improving the health of the local population.

The response from BACCH was the publication of the "Family Friendly Framework" in 2011 which illustrated how services should be commissioned, delivered and improved based on pathways and networks and then this was complemented by the BACCH prospectus in 2012, which provided a detailed description of community child health services including a brief epidemiology of conditions, the role of paediatricians and potential areas for improvement.

2015 and the Future of Community Child Health

The need for "joined-up" integrated thinking has been repeatedly called for over 30 years, especially in the world of child protection/safeguarding, and yet the principal is as equally important for mental health and public health. This remains a challenge which has not yet been successfully overcome, so BACCH produced a paper "The Meaning of Integration for Children and Families" in 2012, in an attempt to create alignment and synergy between commissioners, providers and the interests of CYP.

There continues to be sustained interest in the model of pathways and networks first advocated by BACCH in 1994, and the full potential of such an approach has not yet been researched and embedded throughout clinical services. In order to support more specialist care within community settings, such as disability, mental health and vulnerable childrens' services, community child health departments will have to become larger and/or develop more collaborative approaches with adjacent departments.

Ever better antenatal-neonatal care should improve outcomes, and genetic engineering may reduce the frequency of long-term disabling conditions and be able to predict the likelihood of adult disease earlier in life, but poverty and inequalities and their impact on life course pathways and illness are likely to continue for many years yet and will require proactive public health approaches to both promote and protect the health of the least well resourced in society.

Predicting future morbidity will always be difficult; in 1976 the current concerns of inequalities, ADHD/ASD, obesity and mental health problems were not high on the agenda; today the expectation of perpetual economic growth is not compatible with our planetary ecosystem, and we are beginning to see climate change-related health issues such as extreme weather events and economic migration and in some parts of the world reduction in local food production and emergence of new communicable diseases.

From a health service perspective, future services must be able to adapt more flexibly than they have in the past both to new research and developing technologies, must become more person centric and embrace quality improvement strategies that embed learning within the service delivery.

There is still further potential in developing comprehensive, family-orientated, community-based teams centred on primary care hubs, but with greater expertise, a wider set of competencies and broader skill mix than currently exist. Such a team could reduce unnecessary referrals to hospital and improve the quality of care for those children with long-term conditions.

BACCH will continue to advocate for improved health and health services for children and families throughout the UK for the foreseeable future.

Chairs of CPG/BACCH

1975 Frank Bamford (initial meeting)
1975 Rosemary Graham
1979 Dick Ellis
1983 Neil Gordon
1987 Ross Mitchell
1991 David Baum
1995 Leon Polnay
1999 Jo Sibert
2003 Alan Emond
2007 Nick Spencer
2011 Simon Lenton
2015 Gabrielle Laing

BACCH Affiliated Groups

The *British Academy of Childhood Disability* (BACD) acts as the UK branch of the European Academy of Childhood Disability. www.bacdis.org.uk

The *British Association of Paediatricians in Audiology* (BAPA) former British Association of Community Doctors in Audiology (BACDA). www.bapa.uk.com

The *Child Protection Special Interest Group* (CPSIG): The group works closely with the RCPCH Child Protection Standing Committee. www.cpsig.org.uk

The *British Association for Child and Adolescent Public Health* (previously known as the Child Public Health Interest Group). www.bacaph.org.uk

The *Paediatric Mental Health Association* (PMHA). http://pmha-uk.org/

Ethics

14

Neil McIntosh, Vic Larcher, and Joe Brierley

The three decades covered by this history saw profound changes in public and professional attitudes to severe disability and 'end-of-life' decisions. The paternalistic attitude of an earlier generation was replaced by a welcome move to a more consensual approach, key to which was open discussion with parents, children and young patients. Neil McIntosh, a distinguished neonatologist and professor of child life and health in Edinburgh, was involved in this evolution and the principles established in the report of the College working party he chaired withholding and withdrawing life-sustaining medical treatment, *criticised initially by the medical establishment, have been widely adopted in clinical practice. These form the basis of the present-day guidance, the evolution of which is reviewed by two Great Ormond Street paediatricians, Vic Larcher and Joe Brierley.*

N. McIntosh (✉)
Edinburgh, UK

V. Larcher (✉) • J. Brierley
London, UK

© Springer International Publishing Switzerland 2017
A. Craft, K. Dodd (eds.), *From an Association to a Royal College*,
DOI 10.1007/978-3-319-43582-4_14

The Early Years

Ethics and Terminal Care by Paediatricians and the Ethics Committee: From Leonard Arthur to Withholding and Withdrawing Life-Sustaining Medical Treatment

Neil McIntosh

As a medical student, the apprenticeship of ward teaching was supposed to instil Hippocratic ethics into us as we developed as clinicians. I only vaguely knew what the 'oath' actually said until I heard all the medics at Edinburgh stand, raise their right hands and acknowledge it at their graduations – a moving experience (London medical students were discouraged from physically attending their graduations at the Albert Hall because of the huge numbers involved). In my training years, I worked with senior doctors who oozed skill, experience and good sense. Brompton cocktail and mist euphoria (morphine/cocaine) had been introduced in the late nineteenth century and were used in increasing doses in the management of carcinomatosis and other terminal conditions with us all knowing that this was gradually killing the patient [1]. We took this in our stride and practised it with benevolent paternalism. This paternalism extended to neonatology and paediatrics. In my early days as a registrar, on several occasions, I turned ventilators off in the middle of the night for massive terminal intraventricular haemorrhage and told the mother in the morning, so that she did not have a disturbed night's sleep. How arrogant we were. As a new consultant, this changed to involving the parents in their infant's death, presence and ritual became part of terminal management, but it was our own experience that dictated how and what would happen [2]. It was on this basis that Leonard Arthur hit the headlines in 1980.

Acknowledged as one of the most sensitive paediatricians of his time, he, with the parents' knowledge and sanction and because they did not want their child to survive, prescribed dihydrocodeine 'as required' to reduce the distress of a newborn with Down's syndrome – it took 3 days for the infant to die. He was reported to the police for murder and stood for trial. When he was suspended from work after his first court appearance, a petition with 19,000 signatures, including three Derbyshire MPs, called for his reinstatement. The charge of murder was reduced to attempted murder because the infant was shown to have certain congenital defects. Dr. Arthur did not give evidence himself, but his defence called other distinguished expert witnesses (Sir Douglas Black, president of the Royal College of Physicians, Professor Alex Campbell and Dr. Peter Dunn). The jury, after a trial lasting for many days, deliberated for 2 hours and found Dr. Arthur not guilty.

The case established that it was acceptable to provide 'nursing care only' and confirmed that the administration of a drug by a doctor when necessary to relieve pain is a proper medical practice even when the doctor knows that the drug will itself cause the patient's death – commonly known as the principle of double effect.

The ethics advisory committee of the British Paediatric Association (BPA) was created in 1979. This was in response to the newly developing hospital research ethics committees who were individual often to the point of eccentricity, and many had no conception that children might be different from adults. The committee advised paediatricians who wanted to research with children, offering best practice, initially as outlined by Ross Mitchell [3] and later by the committee itself [4]. Under the chairmanship of Professor Forrester Cockburn and later Professor Alex Campbell, it met infrequently and reactively to matters coming from the way of the paediatricians of the BPA. There is no indication from the association's annual reports that it was asked to comment on the Arthur case.

In the late 1980s, the committee became more proactive and regular in its meetings with lay members in numbers as great as those medical. In 1994 The House of Lords Select Committee on Medical Ethics [5] on taking evidence from the BPA heard that as many as 30 % of neonatal deaths might result from the withdrawal of life-saving medical treatment. In 1996 because of changing views of the public in relation to the medical profession, the committee decided to discuss terminal management, in the context of withholding or withdrawing life-saving medical treatment. Two weekend conferences of those likely to have views were organised at Windsor Castle to take account of legal, moral and ethical perspectives in addition to the formal medical perspective.

In addition to paediatricians working in specialties where such decisions are potentially important (neonatology, neurology, paediatric intensive care, oncology), many others were part of the workshops. We were careful to take advice from people of different religious beliefs (Muslim, Buddhist, Humanist, Jewish and Christian – Jehovah's Witness, Catholic and Protestant). We involved parent groups such as the Stillbirth and Neonatal Death Society and severely handicapped young adults. Nurses-midwives, ethicists and lawyers (both academic and from the Official Solicitors' Office) contributed, and also paediatric surgeons, paediatric anaesthetists and trainee medical and nursing staff working in the areas of concern.

The result of these meetings was *the Withholding and Withdrawal of Life-Saving Medical Treatment – A Framework for Practice* [6]. The document was not meant to be prescriptive, but to outline what was felt to be good practice by those participating. The views were not quite unanimous, one of the five categories to consider causing anxiety for an extremely disabled member of the group, though she accepted them all in principle.

We felt that the five situations where furtherance of life-saving medical treatment might reasonably be considered were:

- The brain-dead child – defined by the usual criteria.
- The persistent vegetative state – a rarity in children.
- The no chance situation – life-sustaining treatment simply delays death, without significant alleviation of suffering.
- The no purpose situation – survival possible with treatment but with a degree of mental and physical impairment that is incompatible with the child in the future taking part in decisions regarding their own treatment or its withdrawal
- The unbearable situation – where the child or family feels that in the face of progressive and irreversible illness, further treatment is more than can be borne.

We emphasised that the decision should be one of a healthcare team (not an individual), and where such a decision was made, this was certainly not an abandonment of the child or family, but that in conjunction with them, there should be a move to more formal palliative care.

Crucial to both editions of the 'framework' are statements that the College and its ethical committee are against euthanasia. Some before [8, 9], and since [10], have pointed out the extremely fine line between the withdrawal of a treatment because of a lack of benefit of that treatment and withdrawal of treatment to ensure the child's death. That death does not always result from withdrawal is clear [11], and parents should be made aware of this prior to withdrawal, with the assurance that full palliative care will be provided for their child. Is withdrawal never carried out to ensure death and what about the use of paralysing agents? These aspects are fully discussed, but when it comes down to it, it is whether or not the paediatrician is being duplicitous in his management of the individual case. As this is rarely if ever an individual decision, but one based on a (usually unanimous) consensus of a healthcare team, there is considerable protection here.

In the paediatric and wider fraternity, the framework has been widely accepted, but however well-made and honourable plans and however general their acceptance, there are always other forces at work. Natural suspicion of authority and genuine paranoia confused with grief can lead down difficult paths for both families and doctors, and the press (sensing extra sales) are always ready to exploit such cases. This occurred for the Leonard Arthur case and even more so and more recently for that of Charlotte Wyatt, where the press were involved early and developed a personal crusade.

Charlotte was born at 26 weeks gestation in Portsmouth weighing only 458 g and after many months of neonatal intensive care had severe chronic lung disease and was believed to be blind and deaf from severe brain damage. It was thought unlikely that she would survive and that her quality of life would be such, if she did, that she would never be able to make any of her own healthcare decisions. Discussion about the withdrawal of life-saving medical treatment with the parents led to an impasse. The staff believed that all they were doing was prolonging an undignified life of pain which had no potential, and the family deciding that all medical care should be applied to their daughter.

The involvement of the papers ensured that the public knew all about the case from the parents' perspective, so the trust felt obliged to seek arbitration in the courts. The case went back and forth. The medical opinion which Mr. Justice Hedley accepted in October 2004 and April 2005 was that it was not in Charlotte's interests to be ventilated in the circumstances set out above. Despite the parents' assurances, in his April 2005 judgement, Mr. Hedley found that there had been no change in Charlotte's underlying condition and that she remained a profoundly disabled baby. In particular, her brain had not grown to any significant extent. After a careful examination of all the arguments for and against ventilation, he decided for the second time that ventilation was not in Charlotte's best interests. The parents appealed but the Court of Appeal concluded that the judge was entitled to continue the declarations.

In the Church of England's contribution to the inquiry, Bishop Butler wrote: 'It may in some circumstances be right to choose to withhold or withdraw treatment, knowing it will possibly, probably, or even certainly result in death'. The church stressed that it was not saying some lives were not worth living but said there were 'strong proportionate reasons' for 'overriding the presupposition that life should be maintained'.

In addition to the newspaper sensationalism, this was the first use of the blogosphere in such a case. Everyone had a view, and many were voiced. The public were at last truly involved in all aspects of medical decision-making in the area.

- I think it's selfish of the parents to want their child to stay alive in constant pain. It's not cruel and unusual to let a child die if that child would pretty much have no future. She can't see or hear. All she knows is pain. Why should they keep her alive? So her parents can keep their child and lose most of their money just trying to keep her breathing?
- Parents should never have to be deprived of their daughter – when something could be done to save her…. Either way, Charlotte should live.
- I think it should be the parent's choice. After all, it is their baby.
- It should be the parent's choice; however, the choice they're making is not the right one to me.
- I think that they should let her go, but the court should not have interfered in my opinion. I'm not a religious person but I do wish them a miracle.
- It should really be the parent's decision, but under the circumstances, I'm going to have to agree with the doctors. It's unethical to keep a child alive that is going through that much pain. It's terrible, but I think that maybe the baby would be better off dead.

Where will we go in the future? In the Netherlands there is carefully managed euthanasia. When I develop my terminal illness in the future, I might go to Switzerland to be put down. My belief is that in any situation, all one can do is the best that one can with firstly all the information available and second with the full involvement of the immediate family members – and sometimes these take time.

Conclusions

Our 'benign paternalism' has moved I think with, rather than because of, the change in society's demands. It has been a difficult road but it makes the individual decisions we are making or recommending no easier. In 1997 the original framework was castigated by the BMA ethics committee – I was summoned to appear before them! Yet about a year later, their own document said almost the same [12]. As Professor the Reverend Gordon Dunstan, the wisest person on our ethics committee, said at the time – 'you can only do your best in these harrowing cases'.

The Post-1997 Era

Vic Larcher and Joe Brierley

The Early Years (1997–2000)

Following the publication of *Withholding and Withdrawal of Life-Saving Medical Treatment – A Framework for Practice* [13], the early years of the RCPCH were active ones for the Ethics Advisory Committee (EAC) and its members. The resolution of several important ethical issues, to which the EAC and its members contributed by the production of policy statements and guidance for members and fellows, helped define the identity of the newly formed college. The ethical issues included subjects as diverse as guidance for the ethical conduct of research with children, recommendations on the acceptance of commercial sponsorship and response to media requests for contact with children. The general approach adopted was one of principled pragmatism. This approach has generally served the College well and has been influential in shaping its ethical perspectives in response to a number of issues that have since arisen. In the case of commercial sponsorship, the approach offered conciliation when other outcomes seemed likely to cause serious differences within the newly formed College.

Guidance for the Ethical Conduct of Research Involving Children (1999)

Guidelines on the ethical conduct of research in children were produced by the Ethics Advisory Committee of the British Paediatric Association in 1980 [4]. Following significant progress in the understanding of children's interests, in legal requirements and in the proper regulation of research, they were revised in 1992 and were further modified and updated by the Royal College of Paediatrics and Child Health in 1999 [14]. They were intended for all involved in the planning, review and conduct of research with children.

The 1999 guidelines were compatible with existing general guidance relating to *all* medical research and were based on these six principles:

1. Research involving children is important for the benefit of all children and should be supported, encouraged and conducted in an ethical manner.
2. Children are not small adults; they have an additional, unique set of interests.
3. Research should only be done on children if comparable research on adults could not answer the same question.
4. A research procedure which is not intended directly to benefit the child subject is not necessarily either unethical or illegal.
5. All proposals involving medical research on children should be submitted to a research ethics committee (REC).
6. Legally valid consent should be obtained from the child, parent or guardian as appropriate. When parental consent is obtained, the agreement of school-age children who take part in research should also be requested by researchers.

Inter alia the document set out criteria for valid worthwhile research in children that included an identifiable prospect of benefit to children, evidence of good scientific and statistical design and avoidance of reduplication; research should not be undertaken primarily for financial or professional advantage; and there should be the intention for proper reporting.

In considering potential benefits, harm and cost, the guidance noted there were no general statutory provisions covering research on human beings. In the absence of such provision, the document offered qualified support for research on children that offered them no direct benefit because absolute protection of children from the potential harms of research denies any of them the potential benefits.

> We therefore support the premise that research that is of no intended benefit to the child subject is not necessarily unethical or illegal. Such research includes observing and measuring normal development, assessing diagnostic methods, the use of "healthy volunteers" and of placebos in controlled trials.

The document acknowledged the importance of evaluating potential benefits, harms and costs of research and the complexity of the task. It outlined the ways in which researchers and reviewers might consider such matters.

Assessments of potential benefits included reviewing estimates of their magnitude, probability, scope (the individual child, the population involved or children in general) and whether the benefits might be limited because of resource considerations. Similarly assessment of harms included their nature, magnitude, probability, timing and future impact, whether it was fair to ask children to face them and what provision might be made if previously unpredicted harms were identified during the course of research. The document also identified the personal and individual nature of harms and the importance of the context in which they occurred. It discussed the classification of risks (the harm involved and the likelihood of its occurrence), classifying them as minimal, low or high, and gave examples of each.

It addressed the then controversial issue of blood sampling for research that was of limited direct benefit to the child as follows:

> We believe that research in which children are submitted to more than minimal risk with only slight, uncertain or no benefit to themselves deserves serious ethical consideration. The most common example of such research involves blood sampling. Where children are unable to give consent, by reason of insufficient maturity or understanding, their parents or guardians may consent to the taking of blood for non-therapeutic purposes, provided that they have been given and understand a full explanation of the reasons for blood sampling and have balanced its risk to their child.........
>
> However we believe that it is completely inappropriate to insist on the taking of blood for nontherapeutic reasons if a child indicates either significant unwillingness before the start or significant stress during the procedure.

The nature, role and purpose of research ethics committees (RECs) were defined, but the responsibilities of *all* concerned in balancing benefits and harms were acknowledged:

> As assessment of benefit and harm is complex. Children are best protected if projects are reviewed at many levels, by researchers, funding and scientific bodies, research ethics

committees, the research assistants and nurses working with child subjects, the children, and their parents. Everyone concerned (except young children) has some responsibility.

Finally the matters of consent (the positive agreement of a person), `assent' (positive acquiescence) and refusal were addressed, as was the general applicability to the concept of Gillick competence as related to research. In terms of a child's refusal:

A reasoned refusal by a child to participate in research is likely to be taken as evidence of such understanding [Gillick competence], and it would be unwise to rely on parental consent in such circumstances.

The guidance contained in the document proved helpful for researchers and reviewers alike in achieving a balance between the protection of research subjects and the facilitation of ethically and scientifically valid research. It was radical in that it recognised the importance of children's consent, involvement in agreement (assent) and refusal and in its approach to so-called nontherapeutic research. It was widely cited and became recognised educational and training material for RECs and researchers alike. Crucially, it presaged the wider involvement of children in the design, conduct and prioritisation of research as set out in the update of 2014 and the Nuffield Council's 2015 report on clinical research with children (see below).

Commercial Sponsorship and the College (1999)

Many organisations, especially those with limited income streams, face difficulties in funding all their desired corporate activities, and the nascent RCPCH was no exception. Sponsorship by companies or individuals can provide much-needed finance – and some types of academic research activity are heavily dependent on sponsorship – but acceptance can produce ethical tensions. Some of these relate to a perception (by both the general public and members of the sponsored organisation) that the organisation accepting sponsorship endorses the aims, activities and products of the sponsor. Some sponsors' activities arouse moral disquiet, and this was the case with the manufacturers of breast-milk substitutes and their sponsorship of BPA and RCPCH activities in the 1990s.

Though recognised as essential for those mothers who cannot or choose not to breast-feed their infants, breast-milk substitutes are considered potentially unsafe and unethical options to breast-feeding in those parts of the world where there is insufficient infrastructure to support their safe use. In 1981 the WHO produced a code concerning the sale and promotion of breast-milk substitutes. The BPA strongly endorsed the code and breast-feeding initiatives. There were concerns that some companies which gave financial support to BPA/RCPCH activities, e.g. the annual meeting, were in breach of the code. Accordingly the BPA held a referendum in 1994 on the question as to whether sponsorship by manufacturers of breast-milk substitutes should continue to be accepted by the organisation. Approximately two-thirds of members voted and of those who did 73 % voted in favour of continued acceptance, with 26.1 % against. Although a 5-year moratorium against debating the issue was imposed by BPA Council, the matter continued to divide the newly formed College. A motion was submitted to the annual meeting of 1997 requesting once again that sponsorship of the

College by milk companies should cease and that the College should seek expert opinion on defining criteria for ethical sponsorship to inform future activities. In the event an amendment was passed which reaffirmed the RCPCH's support of the code, its commitment to develop a strategy to support breast-feeding and instructed the EAC to `consider the broad issues of industrial sponsorship and to draft a definitive College policy document on our relations with industry'.

A working party was convened under the chairmanship of the late Professor David Harvey. It met on 5 occasions and received written and oral submissions from individuals and organisations including researchers, those opposing sponsorship and representatives of infant milk manufactures. A report with 14 recommendations was issued in March 1999 [15] and subsequently endorsed by RCPCH Executive Committee.

The report listed and considered arguments for and against sponsorship and acknowledged the increasing role that it might have in supporting activities that could not attract alternative funding. The approach adopted was one of principled pragmatism, and a distinction was drawn between acceptance of sponsorship of activities of individual members and fellows and that of corporate activities of the College. An absolute ban of all forms of sponsorship was felt to be neither realistic nor practically sustainable, given the financial pressure that would impede the College in attaining its aims and objectives in supporting research that promoted the health and wellbeing of children worldwide if this stance were adopted.

The guiding principle adopted was that the College should not accept sponsorship from organisations and companies whose aims and objectives, as identified by their products or their techniques in promoting them, were incompatible with those of the College. There was – and remains – an absolute embargo on accepting sponsorship from companies that manufacture arms and tobacco or that exploit children. At the time of publication, the position with regard to manufacturers of sugary drinks, alcohol or junk foods was more equivocal though this would be unlikely to be the case today. Sponsorship of general college activities by breast-milk substitute manufacturers was deemed unacceptable although sponsorship of some defined educational, training and research activities was permitted.

Inevitably this proposal was viewed as the compromise it was, but it did offer members and fellows the opportunity to opt out of sponsored activities to which they had moral objections. The formation of a College sponsorship advisory monitoring group to review sponsor applications to the RCPCH went some way to allaying concerns. Moreover there were recommendations that all sources of College sponsorship should be identifiable, transparent and accountable. The College should issue disclaimers to the effect that any acceptance of sponsorship did not imply endorsement of a company or its products.

Acceptance of sponsorship by individual members and fellows or research groups was considered as a matter for individual or collective conscience, subject to the same absolute constraints. The recommended guiding principle was an affirmative response to the question `would you be happy for it to be generally known that you were receiving sponsorship of this type and amount and from this source for this activity?' For researchers there was a recommendation that such research should be under full control of the researcher with free and unfettered publication; it would be wise for research groups where possible to diversify their sources of sponsorship.

At the time the guidance was unique amongst Royal Colleges. It has become more important over time as financial pressures have increased and funding activities became harder. Its recommendations remain core components of the current College sponsorship framework of 2015 [16].

Responses to Media Requests for Contact with and/or Enquiries About Children

The 1990s saw increasing media interest in children and their wellbeing. There was an expansion in visual media platforms and a growing public appetite for human interest stories, especially those in which controversy existed. Not all professionals were happy with this approach, and some had concerns as to what codes of practice governed media personnel and how rigorously they were applied. They were concerned to strike the right balance between the protection of children and families and the legitimate need of the public to be informed and educated on matters concerning the health and wellbeing of children. There was little specific guidance available other than the generic usually brief guidance offered by statutory bodies and defence organisations.

The EAC produced more detailed guidance for professionals on dealing with media requests [17]. It emphasised the need for detailed recording of conversations with media personnel, the avoidance of precipitate and ill-considered disclosure and the need to inform the professional's administration services of the request. For simple requests for brief contacts or interviews, the guidance stressed the importance of informed consent, respect for confidentiality and right of children and families to withdraw at any time.

For more complex projects, involving medium- or long-term involvement or in-depth involvement, the essence of the recommendation was that the proposal should be reviewed before commencement with all the rigour that would be required for ethical review of a research proposal. Matters to be covered included the background to the project, its nature intention and disclosure of conflicts of interests; the expertise and experience of the media personnel involved proof of adherence to media code of practice and valid CRB checks; details of the project itself including a harm-benefits analysis and the time commitment; the procedures for obtaining consent, honouring refusal and respecting confidentiality; any commercial interests involved including insurance matters; and administrative matters, e.g. resource implications and size and impact of production team.

These guiding principles, though never formally updated, have presumably been considered in relation to the production of documentaries about children's hospitals on children's health and behaviours that have been produced over the past decade.

2001–2010

A Decade of Consolidation and Development

After the initial contributions made by the EAC to the establishment of the RCPCH, the subsequent decade was one of consolidation and development for the EAC, with a later incorporation of law into its title and terms of reference so as to better reflect the symbiotic nature of ethics and law in the College.

From Ethics Forum to Ethics and Law Session at the Annual Meeting

An evening ethics forum had been a popular feature of the BPA's annual meeting in York. It was usually case focussed and attracted a wide audience. Its popularity led to the suggestion that there should be a designated half-day ethics and law session, and this occurred from 2000 onwards. Ultimately the responsibility for the organisation of the session was devolved to the Ethics and Law Advisory Committee. Over time competing events affected the numbers attending the evening forum and it was eventually discontinued. The format of the half-day session has varied with guest lectures, interactive sessions, debates and oral and poster presentations, all being used. Joint sessions have been held with palliative care, disability, PICU, etc. Numbers attending have generally been reasonable for group sessions (variably ca 50–60; more on occasions) and feedback largely positive.

Involvement of Children and Young People

As part of the initiative to involve children and young people in the work of the College, the ELAC has encouraged representatives of the young people's forum to attend its meetings to provide input and updates. A formal debate of the motion `This House believes that we have gone too far in granting young people the responsibility for making decisions about their own health care' was held at the annual meeting in 2009 with young people acting as proposers and opposers of the motion and taking an active part in the debate that followed. The proceedings were published in Archives of Disease in Childhood in 2009 [18].

Response to Requests for Consultation

The EAC and latter ELAC have responded to requests made by college officers and EC for input to a wide range of consultations from a variety of bodies ranging from government departments to statutory bodies, e.g. NICE and GMC; topics have included assisted dying, the scope of NICE guidance, children on reality TV shows and pandemic influenza. EAC also considered the training requirements for SpRs in ethics and the law in relation to children.

The Relationship Between Ethics and Law

The EACs were mindful of the sometimes complex interrelationship between medical law and ethics, and the availability of high-quality legal advice was essential in drafting some of the original 1997 and 1999 documents; EAC also recognised the increasing part played by law in matters relating to the care of children in which there is also an ethical dimension, e.g. the UK Human Rights Act 1998, Mental Capacity Act 2005 and Equality Act (and preceding Disability Acts) 2010. EACs were also cognisant of the ethical impact of common law decisions. It was therefore logical for EAC to include law in its title and for its terms of reference to be amended accordingly. The EAC formally became the Ethics and Law Advisory Committee (ELAC) during the decade.

Update of Previous Guidance and Development of New Guidance

In 2004 EAC produced a second edition of *Withholding and withdrawing life-sustaining treatment* [7]. Whilst the basic format and principles underpinning it remained unchanged, the document reflected the emerging role of palliative care in these challenging circumstances.

Responsibilities of Doctors in Child protection Cases with regard to Confidentiality [19] was produced in response to concerns and uncertainties expressed by doctors in relation to disclosure of information in cases where there was good reason to suspect that children had been the subject of abuse or neglect. The document clarified the doctors' primary duties to the child and the legal position with regard to what information should be disclosed and to whom it should be disclosed. Its recommendations have subsequently been incorporated into other RCPCH publications on safeguarding and disclosure.

The Second Decade (2010–Present):

Reviews and Revisions

The two major documents produced by EAC in the early years of the College on *Guidance for the ethical conduct of research involving children* and *Withholding and withdrawing life-sustaining treatment in children: A framework for practice* had served it well, but by the College's second decade, there was an increasing view that revision and review were necessary.

Guidance on Clinical Research Involving Infants, Children and Young People: An Update for Researchers and Research Ethics Committees

A number of factors drove the need to revise the original guidance. These included considerations of the wider-ranging nature of research, e.g. increasing the use of qualitative methodology and changing context in which it occurred, e.g. greater globalisation. The European Clinical Trials Directive 2001/20/EC [19], though applying to less than 13 % of UK research, had legal impact. Over time social and cultural concepts of childhood had evolved to place greater emphasis on children's participation in all aspects of healthcare and research. Finally there was greater acknowledgement of risks of not carrying out research and the resultant harms of inappropriate treatments. There was a sense that the balance between protecting children by viewing them as vulnerable subjects was running counter to their interest and that a more facilitatory approach recognising the scientific importance of ethical research was necessary.

Accordingly a multidisciplinary working party was established and published its recommendations in 2014 [20]. It was branded as 'update' for researchers and RECs. There was no change to underpinning principles, but their interpretation was more facilitatory and reflected the increased need for evidence-based treatment. A new emphasis was on the general obligation to minimise risk with a greater acceptance of quantification of risk in relation to contextual factors. The document had a greater emphasis on scenarios and research in certain specific situations, e.g. palliative care and pregnancy, than the previous generic document. Finally there was further clarification of terms and their implications, e.g. assent was defined as active affirmative agreement; dissent (request to withdraw/refusal of consent) should be respected, but may not be determinative.

Both this and the previous document set the background to the more comprehensive Nuffield Council on Bioethics report on clinical research with children in 2015 [22] which emphasised the importance of children's active participation in the prioritisation, review and implementation of research in striking a balance between facilitation and protection.

Making Decisions to Limit Treatment in Life-Limiting and Life-Threatening Conditions in Children: A Framework for Practice (2015)

There was perhaps a greater need for the review and revision of the original *Withholding and withdrawing life-sustaining treatment in children* document. The pace of change in medical practice had quickened, and there were greater expectations as to what could be delivered and greater use of information technology by parents. The UK had become more socially and culturally diverse. The use of some practices, e.g. the use of muscle relaxants to treat distressing end-of-life symptoms, required greater clarification. The scope of palliative care options had increased, and some treatments, formerly regarded as invasive, were now more widely used as palliation. Both statute law and common law had evolved, and there was an overall sense that change was due.

Although the full procedures that preceded the original document were not duplicated, there were two cycles of consultation with relevant agencies and revision prior to the publication of the final version in 2015. The document was published as a special supplement to the Archives of Disease in Childhood in May 2015, the first occasion on which this had happened for a college document [23].

Notably, the original structure and key ethical principles of the original were retained. In particular the document sets out circumstances under which withholding or withdrawing life-sustaining treatment (LST) might be ethically permissible – NOT circumstances under which such treatment *must* certainly be withheld or withdrawn. It describes situations in which individual children should be spared inappropriate invasive procedures – NOT *types* of children to whom *appropriate* procedures should be denied. The section on palliative care was expanded and that on the child with disabilities clarified and brought into line with current equality legislation.

The document included definitions of key terms and a resume of current practice. The ethical framework included revised consideration of the interests of the child, parental responsibilities and professional duties and factors involved in considering best interests. The process of decision-making section included specific reference to confronting uncertainty, the spectrum of decisions and parental discretion, practical management of end-of-life care and resolution of conflicts. In contrast to the original framework document, three situations were identified when it would be appropriate to consider withholding withdrawal or limitation of life-sustaining treatments because it was no longer in the child's best interests to continue. These were:

1. *When life is limited in quantity (treatment unable or unlikely to prolong life significantly)*
   A. Brain stem death, as determined by agreed professional criteria appropriately applied
   B. Imminent death, where physiological deterioration is occurring irrespective of treatment
   C. Inevitable death, where death is not immediately imminent but will follow and where prolongation of life by LST confers no overall benefit.
2. *When life is limited in quality (treatment may prolong life but not alleviate burdens of disease or treatment)*
   These comprise:
   A. Burdens of treatments, where the treatments themselves produce sufficient pain and suffering so as to outweigh any potential or actual benefits.
   B. Burdens of the child's underlying condition. Here the severity and impact of the child's underlying condition are in itself sufficient to produce such pain and distress as to overcome any potential or actual benefits in sustaining life.
   C. Lack of ability to benefit; the severity of the child's condition is such that it is difficult or impossible for them to derive benefit from continued life.
3. *Informed competent refusal of treatment*
   Adults, who have the capacity to make their own decisions, have the right to refuse LST and to have that refusal respected. So an older child with extensive experience of illness may repeatedly and competently consent to the withdrawal or withholding of life-sustaining treatment. In these circumstances and where the child is supported by his or her parents and by the clinical team, there is no ethical obligation to provide life-sustaining treatment.

The document also included expanded sections on disability, the role of palliative care and ethical review and provided clarification for some specific controversial issues, e.g. the use of muscle relaxants, clinically assisted nutrition and hydration. There was a formal prepublication launch at the Science Media Centre in London.

Quo Vadis: Where Next?

Child health has changed dramatically in the last decade: shared decision-making is the norm, albeit with occasional concern about the diminished professional component and even suggestions for a return to a more (weakly) paternalist approach. Increasingly aggressive technologies in hospital and in children's homes have transformed the landscape with more children than ever living with life-limiting conditions through childhood. The succession of ELAC framework documents has both recognised and anticipated these changes.

The ELAC continues to evolve and in more recent years it has worked with a number of other bodies. Thus it has provided members for the Nuffield Council on Bioethics Working Party that produced Children and Clinical Research: Ethical Issues; the recent DH Ebola Communications and Engagement Stakeholder Group; and the DH UK Donation Ethics committee. ELAC now has a standing member from the Royal College of Nursing in recognition of the nurse's fundamental role in all aspects of child health and members of the RCPCH EC as standing members, in recognition of the important role the ELAC plays in daily college business.

Responses to various consultations about possible opening up of the Family Division of the High Court, ethical reviews of cosmetic surgery and assisted dying have recently been produced. As well as this reactive role members of ELAC have also been proactive in calling for the formation of the RCPCH Working Party that reviewed and amended the clinical guidance of verification of death in infancy. They have argued for the provision of training workshops on elements of its published guidance for the College and others and actively contributed to these events. In recognition of the crucial role the media play in child health, the ELAC provides regular support to the RCPCH communications and media team including `horizon scanning' about emerging topics of importance.

This more proactive stance will soon be reflected in the formation of a new RCPCH Children's Ethics and Law Special Interest Group (CHELSIG) which will be open to all professional groups and take over provision of the Ethics and Law Forum/content for the Annual Conference, enable a multidisciplinary open forum for all those interested in the ethical and legal issues affecting children and enable and support an academic backdrop to infant, child and young people's ethics and law. Thus CHELSIG should be ideally placed to analyse and reflect upon the ethical issues that impact on the lives of children and their families in the wider healthcare setting and provide informed debate and opinion in these areas. The intention is that CHELSIG will interact fluidly with ELAC, but will have a wider role by interfacing actively with other relevant bodies such as children's hospital ethics committees and national and international specialist society ethics groups whilst leaving the ELAC, itself, to focus on being the elected Ethics and Law Advisory entity for the RCPCH.

Coda

Time will tell whether the revision of the two key documents alluded to will prove as helpful as the originals. That the originals withstood the test of time is a tacit acknowledgement to the integrity and intellectual rigour of the principles that underpinned them. They underscore the importance of sound ethical foundations to the future aims and objectives of the College. ELAC will continue to support college members, children and families and, via CHELSIG, more broadly other professionals involved in child health.

References

The Early Years

1. Snow H. Opium and cocaine in the treatment of cancerous disease. Br Med J. 1896;ii:718–9.
2. McIntosh N, Eldridge C. Neonatal death – the neglected side of neonatal care? Arch Dis Child. 1984;59:585–7.
3. Mitchell R. The child and experimental medicine. Br Med J. 1964;i:721–7.
4. British Paediatric Association Working Party on Ethics of Research on Children. Guidelines to aid ethical committees considering research involving children. Arch Dis Child. 1980;55: 75–7.
5. Report of the House of Lords Select Committee on Medical Ethics, House of Lords. 1994;1:47.
6. RCPCH Ethics Advisory Committee. Withholding and with drawing life-saving medical treatment. A framework for practice. RCPCH, London; 1997.
7. RCPCH Ethics Advisory Committee. Withholding and withdrawing life sustaining medical treatment. A framework for practice. RCPCH, London;2004.
8. Anonymous. 'Points of View'. Non-treatment of defective newborn babies. Lancet. 1979;314: 1123–4.
9. Brereton RJ. Severe handicap in the newborn: treatment, non-treatment or assisted death. Lancet. 1979;314:1372.
10. Silverman WA. Compassion or opportunism. Pediatrics. 2004;113:402.
11. Balfour-Lynn IM, Tasker RC. Futility and death in paediatric medical intensive care. J Med Ethics. 1996;22:279–81.
12. BMA Ethics Committee. Withholding and withdrawing life prolonging medical treatment. Guidance for decision making. BMA publications. RCPCH, London; 1999.

The Post-1997 Era

13. RCPCH Ethics Advisory Committee. Withholding and withdrawing life-saving medical treatment. A framework for practice. RCPCH, London; 1997.
14. RCPCH. Ethics advisory committee and professor David Hull guidelines for the ethical conduct of medical research involving children. Arch Dis Child. 2000;82:177–82.
15. Commercial sponsorship in the RCPCH, Report of a Working Party 1999 (Chair: Professor David Harvey) (http://www.rcpch.ac.uk/sites/default/files/asset_library/Publications/C/Commercial%20 Sponsorship%20in%20the%20Royal%20College%20of%20Paediatrics%20and%20Child%20 Health.pdf).
16. RCPCH sponsorship framework of 2015(ratified by RCPCH Council April 2015). RCPCH/07/15.
17. RCPCH Ethics Advisory Committee. Advice to paediatricians and other professionals in responses to media requests for contact with and/or enquiries about children; A guidance note RCPCH. 1999.
18. Larcher V, Elias-Jones A, Mepani B, Brierley J. "This House believes that we have gone too far in granting young people the responsibility for making decisions about their own health care". A record of a debate held in the Ethics and Law session of the RCPCH Annual Meeting York 2009. Arch Dis Child. 2011;96:123–6.
19. RCPCH Responsibilities of doctors in child protection with regard to confidentiality. RCPCH, London; 2004.

20. Medicines for Human Use (Clinical Trials) Regulations. 2004. www.legislation.hmso.gov.uk/si/si2004/20041031.htm. http://www.wma.net/en/30publications/10policies/b3/.
21. Modi N, Vohra J, Preston J, Elliott C, Van't Hoff W, Coad J, Gibson F, Partridge L, Brierley J, Larcher V, Greenough A, Working Party of the Royal College of Paediatrics and Child Health. Guidance on clinical research involving infants, children and young people: an update for researchers and research ethics committees. Arch Dis Child. 2014;99:887–91.
22. Nuffield Council on Bioethics. Children and clinical research: ethical issues Nuffield Council on Bioethics. 2015. ISBN 978-1-904384-31-1http://nuffieldbioethics.org/wp-content/uploads/Children-and-clinical-research-full-report.pdf.
23. Larcher V, Craig F, Bhogal K, Wilkinson D, Brierley J. Making decisions to limit treatment in life-limiting and life-threatening conditions in children: a framework for practice. Arch Dis Child. 2015;100 Suppl 2:s1–26. doi:10.1136/archdischild-2014-306666.

Research

15

Anne Greenough

Research has always been an important part of improving the health and welfare of children. There are many academic departments of paediatrics which undertake vitally important and ground breaking work. In addition there are some issues which are best addressed at something more than a local level and the BPA then the College have taken the lead in areas of research which are best tackeld utilising the unique resources of the College Membership. Anne Greenhough is the current Vice President for research and here recounts the development of this important College function.

The Research Unit was established in 1994, but its origins were over 10 years earlier when the BPA recruited staff to assist with the biennial workforce census and other surveys. By 1993 the need for research and information had grown to the extent that the President David Hull proposed the establishment of a dedicated Research Unit. Terms of reference for the new unit, which were approved in October 1994, set out the aims of initiating and facilitating new research, with a guiding principle that this should have a national perspective and that the unit should not compete with academic departments or be a financial drain on the college or its members. A grant of £60,000 from Nestle was secured to establish the unit, which lead to a heated debate within the BPA membership about the rights and wrongs of taking commercial sponsorship from baby milk manufacturers and resulted eventually in the formation of an Ethics Advisory Committee when the RCPCH was founded.

The newly established unit was led by the Director, Professor David Baum, and a Principal Research Officer, Dr Jon Pollock, was appointed to manage the staff team. From the outset it was agreed that the BPSU should be affiliated to the Research Unit and over the next few years the work of other BPA committees was gradually incorporated. By 1996, the work included health services research,

A. Greenough
London, UK

© Springer International Publishing Switzerland 2017
A. Craft, K. Dodd (eds.), *From an Association to a Royal College*,
DOI 10.1007/978-3-319-43582-4_15

national clinical audit, the workforce census and, from 1997, the work of a Paediatric Formulary Committee developing the paediatric formulary Medicines for Children.

Research projects undertaken in these early years included Department of Health-funded research into the screening and management of retinopathy of prematurity and a confidential enquiry into the healthcare delivery and outcomes of meningococcal disease funded by the Meningitis Research Foundation and the National Lottery. Membership support and advice was also an important function with research workshops at the Annual Scientific Meeting and guides to funding sources and information about children's health. By 1998, when David Baum became President, the Research Unit had evolved into a department of research and information, encompassing the surveillance of rare diseases, health services research and audit work.

When the college was formed in 1996, responsibility for the Research Unit had been incorporated into the portfolio of the Vice President for Science and Research, and in 1998 Professor Richard Cooke became director. Shortly afterwards, the unit became the Research Division and when Jon Pollock left the college, Linda Haines became the Principal Research Officer. Over the next few years, successes in national funding rounds continued, with projects such as a National Lottery-funded project on chronic fatigue syndrome. During this time, the discipline of evidence-based practice was becoming increasingly important, and in 1999 the Quality of Practice Committee was brought within the Research Division and the programme expanded to include the dissemination of evidence-based guidance and CHERUB, a monthly evidence bulletin for members.

In 2002 Professor Neil McIntosh became Vice President for Science and Research and under his leadership an important new programme on child protection began. In 2003 a survey of members about complaints achieved an exceptionally high response and generated significant press interest and led to a college-wide programme to support doctors working in child protection. Related Research Division projects included qualitative studies with paediatricians and parents. In 2005 a joint project with the Advocacy Committee and Parents and Carers liaison group exploring how children and young people could participate in the work of the college resulted in the publication 'Coming out of the Shadows' which made recommendations to the college about children's participation. Around this time concerns about an epidemic of childhood obesity led to the establishment of a group to identify research priorities. The outcome was a BPSU study on type 2 diabetes and a project on interventions to prevent high-risk infants from developing obesity runs from the University of Warwick.

In 2003 the Research Division began to develop clinical practice guidelines in areas where research had identified a specific need. Thus the first RCPCH guideline was on CFS/ME, and this was followed by an RCPCH/RCOphth guideline on Screening and Treatment of Retinopathy of Prematurity in 2007. In 2006 the project to update and evidence base the Royal College of Physicians' publication on the physical signs of child sexual abuse began, and this resulted in an important updated publication (Chap. 17). However by the time the guideline on hypernatraemia had been completed in 2010, the focus had moved from guideline development to ensuring wider paediatric involvement in NICE guidance. In 2005 the division was relocated to Great Portland Street to accommodate the satellite unit of the NICE Women and Children's Collaborating Centre to facilitate closer working relationships. Although this group moved out in 2006, the Research Division remained there until it moved to Theobalds Road in 2009.

In 2007 Professor Terence Stephenson took over responsibility for the Research Division before becoming President in 2009. During this period the Division's reputation led to four projects being commissioned by the Department of Health. These included a national survey (2009) to establish the number of children with diabetes and the development of new UK growth charts for children 0–5 years. This high-profile project was delivered in a very short time and meant that the UK was the first country to incorporate the WHO growth standard. Other DH-funded projects were the project to establish the care pathway of children with feverish illness, led by the Clinical Effectiveness Team, and a project to develop evidence-based care pathways for children with allergies.

In April 2009 Professor Neena Modi became Vice President for Science and Research and soon after the Research Division became a department of a broader Directorate in a college-wide restructure. Under her guidance, college research continued to thrive, with important national audits on neonatal care, diabetes and epilepsy. The RCPCH continues to undertake important national audits in neonatal care, diabetes and now stroke. The department also bids successfully to obtain the funding for national reviews of mortality and morbidity in children. The NHS reforms for England saw the disappearance of the National Patient Safety Agency, and the Research Department has taken over responsibility for highlighting safety concerns for children and young people in England's NHS.

The BPA first published guidance in relation to research involving children in 1980. That guidance initiated a sea change stating 'research involving children is important', 'should be supported and encouraged' and 'research which involves a child and is of no benefit to that child (nontherapeutic research) is not necessarily unethical or illegal'. This has most recently been updated in 2014. The working party involved representatives from the Royal College of Nursing, the Ethics and the Law Advisory Committee of the RCPCH, the National Research Ethics Service, the Medicines and Healthcare Regulatory Agency, the General Medical Council, the Medical Research Council, WellChild, the Medicines for Children Research Network (MCRN), the NIHR Paediatrics (non-medicines) Specialty Group and the NIHR MCRN Young Person's Advisory Group. The report highlighted that regulation, whilst providing protection for participants and researchers alike and consistency of processes, is also crucial to benefit health and well-being through facilitation of high-quality research. The greater involvement of young people in all aspects of research was documented and commended. Parents, children and young people have a vital role to play in advocating for research. This is being taken forward by the RCPCH's & Us and the NIHR's Generation R. The RCPCH is developing a Children and Young People's Research Charter.

Professor Modi as VP Science and Research led a working group to better understand the challenges of undertaking child health research. The report 'Turning the Tide: Harnessing the Power of Child Health Research' published in 2013 made a number of recommendations including the need to recognise the relevance of children's research, not only to their health and well-being but also to that of the nation and successive generations. The report drew attention to the potential of early year's research being harnessed but required a long vision and a resourced strategy that has as its metric the health of the nation. The report highlighted that although the NIHR Integrated Academic Training Programme attracted high-calibre paediatricians, children's research groups in general lacked critical mass. In addition, a major impediment to progress was inadequacies in opportunities for trainees to be exposed to research and acquire core research skills and knowledge of research regulation and governance. Turning the Tide highlighted that funding of child health research is challenging as only one national children's research charity had a research spend exceeding £1.5 million per annum, largely precluding their ability to support large clinical trials and major research programmes, establish substantive research posts or fund infrastructure. The RCPCH, therefore, provided the infrastructure to develop the UK Child Health Research Collaboration where UK child health research charities come together. The aims of UKCHRC include working towards collaborative solutions to generic problems in child health research and facilitate partnership funding of larger projects.

Subsequently, Anne Greenough (VP Science and Research) has established a research strategy collaboration committee involving the four devolved nations, funders, CYP, academic trainees and academics, and a committee of the research leads the Children's Speciality Groups and the NIHR Clinical Study Groups to inform the RCPCH's research priorities and provide a resource to give timely and well-informed expert opinions on research issues.

From 1999 onwards the research division has carried out a biennial workforce census providing essential evidence to support RCPCH health policy. In response to health service reorganisations and the introduction of working time regulations, workforce assessment at the RCPCH has expanded to include studies about the impact of EWTD, the benefits of consultant-delivered care and regular reports on rota compliance and vacancies. Annual studies of trainees career intentions, research capacity and outcomes for new CST holders have meant the RCPCH has a crucial influence on workforce planning decisions in all four UK nations. Most recently, a survey of members in 2015 highlighted a further reduction in research-active paediatricians. As a consequence, a pilot scheme has been undertaken between BAPM and the RCPCH to introduce research training for all trainees with the aim of rolling this out to all speciality groups. In addition, a database of research funding opportunities has been established for all RCPCH members informed by the members of UKCHRC.

All of the vice presidents who oversaw the research portfolio were college officers with full-time busy academic jobs in the universities which employed them. The department would never have enjoyed the very considerable success over two decades without the tireless work of the staff who did the hard yards, day to day. The college has been very fortunate to see those staff led over that time initially by Dr Jon Pollock and then until 2010 by Linda Haines. In January 2011 the Research Department became incorporated into a new Directorate of Research and Policy where the good work has continued under the leadership of Jacqueline Fitzgerald.

The British Paediatric Surveillance Unit (BPSU)

16

Euan Ross, Richard Lynn, and Richard Reading

Rare diseases and infections are by definition individually uncommon, but collectively they are an important cause of morbidity and mortality in childhood. With that in mind, the British Paediatric Surveillance Unit (BPSU) was set up in 1986 to address this. Through the simple methodology of circulating monthly report cards, the Unit has enabled paediatricians in the UK and Eire to participate in the surveillance and further study of uncommon disorders affecting children. After 30 years of continuous active surveillance, the BPSU has facilitated over 100 studies leading to over 300 scientific publications. The unit is regarded as a major British contributor to practical medical epidemiology.

History

The BPSU arose from a number of pressures operating in the early 1980s. Whilst the then British Paediatric Association (BPA) was growing rapidly through consultant expansion, simultaneously the Communicable Disease Surveillance Centre (CDSC) of the Public Health Laboratory Service (PHLS) in London, headed by Dr Spence Galbraith, wished to develop a system to speedily

E. Ross • R. Lynn
London, UK

R. Reading (✉)
Norwich, UK

© Springer International Publishing Switzerland 2017
A. Craft, K. Dodd (eds.), *From an Association to a Royal College*,
DOI 10.1007/978-3-319-43582-4_16

recognise and monitor newly recognised infectious disease. Galbraith (rightly) surmised that paediatricians would be a fruitful group to approach. There was good reason to believe this. Paediatricians had already been involved in a card reporting system in the 1960s when helping to collect data for a study of lead poisoning encephalopathy, undertaken by Professor David Barltrop and colleagues at St Mary's Hospital. This methodology was adopted by the National Childhood Encephalopathy Study codirected by Professor David Miller and Dr Euan Ross at the Middlesex Hospital Medical School. In the course of 3 years, consultant paediatricians reported 1182 cases of infant encephalopathic disease.

The early 1980s saw passive reporting of Reye's syndrome, haemolytic uraemic syndrome, Kawasaki disease and haemorrhagic shock encephalopathy syndrome by paediatricians to CDSC. However, it was felt that under-ascertainment could be occurring so active surveillance was considered.

Discussions were held in 1984 between what were to be the parent bodies of the BPSU: the BPA, PHLS and the Institute of Child Health (London). A small steering committee later to be known as the BPSU Executive Committee (BEC) under the chairmanship of ex-president of the BPA, Sir Peter Tizard, was then set up. Sitting on the BEC were the three parent bodies along with representatives from the Faculty of Paediatrics of the Royal College of Physicians (Ireland) and the then Communicable Disease Surveillance Centre (Scotland). The BEC considered how best to implement active surveillance using the methodologies previously developed. It was felt that the introduction of such a system would allow for the increased ascertainment necessary for assessing trends in rare disorders. Such a system would reduce the number of requests received by clinicians from individual researchers for data.

The objectives of the BPSU were:

- To facilitate research into uncommon childhood disorders for the advancement of knowledge.
- To allow paediatricians to participate in surveillance.
- To increase the awareness within the medical profession and respond rapidly to public health emergencies.
- From the outset it was agreed that simplicity was to be the watch word. The BEC of today still takes these principles to heart.

So it was in July 1986 when the first BPSU orange card was dispatched listing the names of six disorders, AIDS, Lowe syndrome, HUS, neonatal herpes, SSPE and X-linked anhidrotic ectodermal dysplasia to 800 consultant paediatricians in the UK and Ireland.

British Paediatric Surveillance Unit Report Card

NOTHING TO REPORT [   ]   July 1986

Specify in the box number of cases seen   CODE No [ ]

[ ] AIDS
[ ] X-linked anhydrotic ectodermal dysplasia
[ ] Haemorrhagic Shock Encephalopathy Syndrome

[ ] Haemolytic Uraemic Syndrome
[ ] Neonatal Herpes
[ ] Kawasaki Disease
[ ] Reye's Syndrome

[ ] SSPE
[ ]

Governance and Administration

Now, as then, the executive committee consists of paediatricians and clinical epidemiologists drawn from a wide range of the disciplines that make up paediatrics. Much of the original success of the Unit can be laid at the door of Dr Susan Hall, consultant epidemiologist, and Myer Glickman, administrator, who implemented the wishes of the committee. From 1990 the scientific coordinator post has been held by Richard Lynn who, since the early years of this century, has been assisted by a research facilitator. There are two medical advisers who liaise between researchers and the BPSU Committee.

The governance and oversight of the BPSU has continued to be provided by the three parent bodies. The BPA has become the RCPCH, the PHLS in England has become Public Health England (PHE) and the ICH has now been incorporated into the University College London. All three continue to act as parent bodies.

At its outset the BPSU was aware that it could not be a financial burden on its parent bodies. The past President of the Royal College of Physicians, Sir Cyril Clarke, was instrumental in obtaining a grant from an anonymous Trust. A long association with the Children Nationwide Medical Research Fund followed this. From 2006–2009 the Unit was supported by a grant from the DH, who recognised its contribution to public health in the UK. Further funding is raised through an annual fee by each study using the system. The unit also recognises the uncosted contributions of time and effort made by the parent bodies.

By 2012 a funding crisis precipitated a detailed review of the funding and governance of the BPSU. This led to a more active engagement of the three parent bodies, a separation of finance and governance from the scientific work of the BPSU and the establishment of a governance board with representation from the three parent bodies, whilst the executive committee was relaunched as the Scientific Committee (SC) of the BPSU.

The BEC, and subsequently SC, have been chaired successively by the following:

Sir Peter Tizard, David Baum, Euan Ross, Catherine Peckham, Chris Verity, Mike Preece, Allan Colver, Alan Emond and Richard Reading.

Methodology

Each month all consultant and associate specialist paediatricians in the four countries of the UK and the Republic of Ireland are asked to complete a reporting card listing the conditions currently under surveillance. Originally an orange postcard (hence the "orange card") was used, but the reporting is now done electronically. Between 10 and 14 studies are included in the reporting card at any one time. A set of instructions for completing the card, including case definitions of the conditions listed on the card, is also circulated.

Respondents are asked to return the card to the BPSU office, indicating the number of cases of each condition on the card which they have managed during the preceding calendar month. An important feature of the system is the returning of the cards even if no cases are seen, thus allowing us to monitor compliance. Consistently over the years, between 90 % and 95 % of cards are returned. Once the BPSU office is made aware that a clinician has seen a case, the researcher undertaking the appropriate study is informed. They then contact the clinicians to collect the relevant data. Over 90 % of these requests are completed. Since its inception over 25,000 cases have been reported.

The Unit, although initiating some projects, in the main is there to facilitate the research interests of the RCPCH members. Following an initial enquiry, those wishing to place a condition on the card receive a package of information to help them develop an outline proposal. If the developmental proposal sounds suitable for incorporation within the BPSU, a more detailed application is requested. Much of the development of the application is undertaken through discussions with the BEC's medical advisers. Although this iterative process is sometimes criticised for taking a long time, much of this relates to incorporating epidemiological principles such as a robust case definition, and ensuring maximum ascertainment, into a studies which are usually initiated by clinicians who may not have considered the finer points of epidemiology.

Since the early 2000s, the work of the BPSU has been increasingly influenced by the need for public and patient engagement. There have been two lay representatives on the BEC/SC who comment on all applications and who have helped develop guidance and recommendations about public and patient engagement in individual surveillance studies. Whilst patient engagement has become an increasingly prominent feature of all research, the BPSU takes it particularly to heart as it is one way of providing an assurance that the research carried out by the BPSU, which by its nature uses clinical data without consent or knowledge of individual patients, is in the public interest. Other assurances are that all data is subject to strict data security arrangements, and studies need to receive approval from official bodies charged with monitoring use of health data in research (The Confidentiality Advisory Group of the Health Research Authority in England and the Public Benefit and Privacy Panel in Scotland).

Many of the projects come from major academic units but by no means all. The chemistry set poisoning study initiated by Tom Mucklow from the Isle of Wight is but one example of a successful study which contributed to legislation for children's toys.

Achievements

The BPSU has surpassed its original expectations in its achievements. Not only has the unit supported researchers in the study of rare disorders, but also the outcomes have had a substantial impact on public health. As early as 1986, the BPSU was monitoring the effects of new warnings about aspirin and Reye's syndrome. The Unit has kept under surveillance diseases targeted by vaccination programmes as well as late sequelae. Examples include the surveys on congenital rubella, meningo-encephalitis after MMR vaccine, acute flaccid paralysis and Hib vaccine failures, and more recent examples include anaphylaxis after immunisation. The unit has provided the base for reporting HIV and AIDS in children in the UK and Ireland. To achieve this it has cooperated with obstetricians, laboratories and others to give maximum surveillance coverage. Through the BPSU, the dramatic reduction in perinatal transmission of HIV has been documented – one of the public health triumphs of recent years. One of the aims of the Unit is to have a 'rapid response' to emerging public health crises. Here the Unit helped assess the impact of changing the route of administration of vitamin K in newborn infants, following concern about a possible link between vitamin K injections and the subsequent development of childhood cancers. Since 1997 the BPSU has been involved in the monitoring of new variant Creutzfeldt-Jakob disease in children through the Progressive and Intellectual Neurological Disorder (PIND) survey and also the monitoring of *E. coli* 0157 outbreaks and its impact on the level of haemolytic uraemic syndrome in children (three studies – 1986–1989, 1997–2001 and 2010–2014). The 2008 pandemic of swine flu and the subsequent mass vaccination campaign led to concerns about possible Guillain-Barre syndrome as a rare clinical sequel, which was investigated (and refuted) by a BPSU study run in 2009–2010.

Screening and public health policy has been informed by a number of BPSU studies. The current policy on newborn screening for medium-chain acyl-CoA dehydrogenase deficiency (MCAD) was dependent on two BPSU studies into this condition (1994–1996 and 2004–2006). More recently, studies on congenital adrenal hyperplasia have informed screening policy on this condition, whilst a study on congenital hypothyroidism has investigated the yield and outcome of neonatal screening. Two studies on neonatal group B streptococcal infection (2000–2001 and

2014–2015) illustrate how the changing epidemiology of infectious disease can result in different advice about screening and treatment policies in pregnant women.

Further achievements can be seen in the educational role the Unit has played, through the publication of an annual report, a newsletter, over 300 publications and presentations and the holding of national conferences, seminars and workshops. The Unit also now has its own website www.rcpch.ac.uk/bpsu.

Such has been the success of this methodology that it has been adopted by other medical specialities within the UK, including child psychiatry, obstetrics, ophthalmology, neurology, gastroenterology, dermatology and occupational health medicine. In other countries 10 other paediatric surveillance units have been established, from Australia, Germany, Netherlands, Switzerland, Papua New Guinea, Malaysia, New Zealand Latvia, Canada and nearer home Wales, Scotland and Ireland. Many of these units have now linked up to form the International Network of Paediatric Surveillance Units. This network intends to increase communication between researchers, develop standardised research protocols, promote and develop new national units and undertake surveillance on a global basis.

Conclusion

The BPSU started in 1986 sending out its orange reporting card. It is now a well-established part of British paediatric practice and has its part in the history of epidemiology. Over the past three decades, the BPSU has met and exceeded the aims set by its founders principally by sticking to its founding principles of robust simplicity. In maintaining this we have every hope that it will continue to act as a global model for developing child health epidemiology.

As Sir Cyril Clarke said in 1991 'British and Irish paediatricians therefore feel justly proud of themselves as the pioneers and key enactors of this unique reporting system'.

Child Protection and Safeguarding

17

Jo Sibert and Jeff Debelle

The foundation of the College in 1996 coincided with the increasing realisation that child protection was not just the role of a small group of specialist community paediatricians but every paediatrician's responsibility. The investigation of possible abuse to children and its prevention has become an increasingly important part of a paediatrician's everyday work.

This meant that the place of child protection/safeguarding has assumed a much greater role in the life of the College than previously with the BPA. The primary role of the college has been to set and maintain standards and to be responsible for training and examination of doctors, but this has now included making certain that paediatricians have access to the best possible evidence in making the diagnosis of abuse and responding to reports and enquiries into abuse. It has also involved support for paediatricians. All this, of course, takes place within a multi-agency and multidisciplinary context. Prevention is vital in the paediatrician's response to abuse, and in 1994 there was involvement by the National Commission of Enquiry into the prevention of child abuse, and the BPA was represented on this by Jo Sibert.

Organisation

In 1989 the BPA and the British Association of Paediatric Surgeons (BAPS) set up a Joint Standing Committee on Child Abuse (later renamed the Joint Standing Committee for Child Protection), and this has remained the vehicle for the BPA and then the College to respond to the various crises which have hit the profession over the subsequent years. In 2015 this is now the Child Protection Standing Committee,

J. Sibert (✉)
Cardiff, UK

J. Debelle
Birmingham, UK

© Springer International Publishing Switzerland 2017
A. Craft, K. Dodd (eds.), *From an Association to a Royal College*,
DOI 10.1007/978-3-319-43582-4_17

chaired by the officer for child protection, which leads the college input into safeguarding matters. BAPS are no longer involved but there is representation from RCGP, NSPCC, Departments of Health and Education, Child Protection Special Interest Group (CPSIG), Faculty of Legal Medicine of RCP and representatives from the four nations.

The Child Protection Special Interest Group (CPSIG) runs in parallel with the Standing Committee on Child Protection. It was established in the 1980s by paediatricians, including Dr Chris Hobbs and Dr Jane Wynne from Leeds, to provide a forum for those working in the field of child maltreatment. CPSIG is a special interest group of the British Association for Community Child Health (BACCH) and in 2005 was formally recognised as an independent special interest group affiliated to the RCPCH. CPSIG representatives sit on the BACCH Executive and RCPCH standing committee on Child Protection. The CPSIG, along with the Joint Standing Committee, is responsible for safeguarding session at the Annual Conference.

Responding to Reports

Throughout the latter part of the twentieth century, there were a series of high-profile abuse cases, many of which led to national enquiries and recommendations for improvements in the way that the protection of children was handled. The case of Maria Colwell was one of the first, but there have been many more. In the mid-1980s, there was the first recognition that child sexual abuse was a hidden and unrecognised form of abuse. Over a short period of time, two paediatricians in the county of Cleveland diagnosed many children with sexual abuse, and for the majority this was on the basis of a previously unrecognised physical sign of reflex anal dilatation. This episode was hugely controversial with many children being removed from their parents and taken into the care of the local authority. The response of the Government was to set up a committee of enquiry chaired by Dame Elizabeth Butler Sloss, and Professor David Hull, later President of the BPA, was appointed as paediatrician to the enquiry. This led to the Children Act of 1989 and to the Department of Health guidance on the practical aspects of investigating and managing suspected child abuse and its prevention.

Working Together to Protect Children followed in 1989 with the hope that high-profile tragedies would be a thing of the past, but of course they did happen again. The tragic case of Victoria Climbié led to a report by Lord Laming with one of his many findings being a failure of communication between professionals. Once again guidance on this, Working Together to Protect Children, was produced. The RCPCH played its role in responding to these reports. The advice has recently been updated as *Working Together to Safeguard Children* (HM Government, 2015).

Since 2006 there has continued to be a series of reports which have emphasised the need for College involvement in child protection. These documents include:

- Lord Laming's progress report in 2009 on his original report following the death of Victoria Climbié, The Protection of Children in England: Progress Report

- Professor Sir Ian Kennedy's report in 2010, Getting it right for children and young people
- Professor Eileen Munro's review of child protection in 2011 on behalf of the Department for Education, Final Report – A child-centred system
- NICE guidance on child maltreatment in 2009, When to Suspect Child Maltreatment
- Revised statutory guidance in 2013 and 2015, Working Together to Safeguard Children

Sadly controversial child abuse cases still occur as shown by the response to the death of Baby Peter in 2006.

Evidence

One of the key roles of the College was and is to guide paediatricians into the correct diagnosis of abuse. In the late 1990s, there was considerable concern that practice in child protection was not evidence based. This led to a series of systematic reviews from Cardiff led by Alison Kemp, Sabine Maguire and Jo Sibert. This work was funded by the NSPCC with help from the RCPCH and others. This and much other work led to the development of the *Child Protection Companion* by the college in 2006. A second edition was published in June 2013. It emphasised the importance of sharing and co-ordinating care in a multidisciplinary fashion and provides guidance for paediatricians on everything from examination and identification of children presenting with nonaccidental injuries, through referral and court proceedings. It contains information on the latest evidence, research, guidance, publications and standards on child safeguarding. The NSPCC are no longer involved in this work and the College has taken full responsibility for it.

Fabricated or Induced Illness by Carers (FII)

This form of abuse, previously known as Munchausen syndrome by proxy, caused concern within the RCPCH, largely because of several high-profile cases that resulted in the setting up of a working party and the publishing of the first edition of *Fabricated or Induced Illness by Carers* in 2002. In 2009, a further working party chaired by Dr Paul Davis studied the subject and published the second edition as a *Practical Guide* published by the Department of Health. This guidance was confirmed by a review in 2012. One of the key points was the importance of a detailed chronology, and another was the need for a responsible paediatric consultant to oversee the management of the child.

Acute life-threatening events (ALTEs) and those in whom it is thought that there might be imposed upper airway obstruction form part of the spectrum of FII. They are reviewed in both editions of the *Practical Guide*. A report produced by

Frank Bamford and colleagues evaluated the evidence and concluded that such external obstruction of the airways did sometimes take place.

One of the issues arising from the concerns around sudden infant death (SIDs) was the lack of consistency around the country as to how these tragic events were investigated. The College asked Baroness Helena Kennedy to chair a working group who came up with recommendations as to how SIDs should be managed. These were largely taken up and implemented by the Department of Health [Kennedy H, Sudden unexpected Death in Infancy, 2004. RCPCH and RCPath].

The General Medical Council

There is no doubt that the GMC's attitude to paediatricians working in child protection caused much concern amongst many Members and Fellows of the RCPCH. This particularly followed the cases (eventually dismissed) against Professor Sir Roy Meadow and Professor David Southall. In the early part of the twenty-first century, an orchestrated campaign began against those involved in the field of child protection. Paediatricians in particular were targeted and as a consequence many paediatricians were reluctant to get involved in such cases as expert witnesses. In 2004 the College undertook a survey of members, which had an over 80% response rate, and asked whether they had had a complaint against them concerning child protection: 736 complaints had been received by 565 doctors. The vast majority of these were investigated and dismissed but nevertheless made paediatricians reluctant to get involved in child protection, and lawyers were having great difficulty finding experts for the necessary expert work.

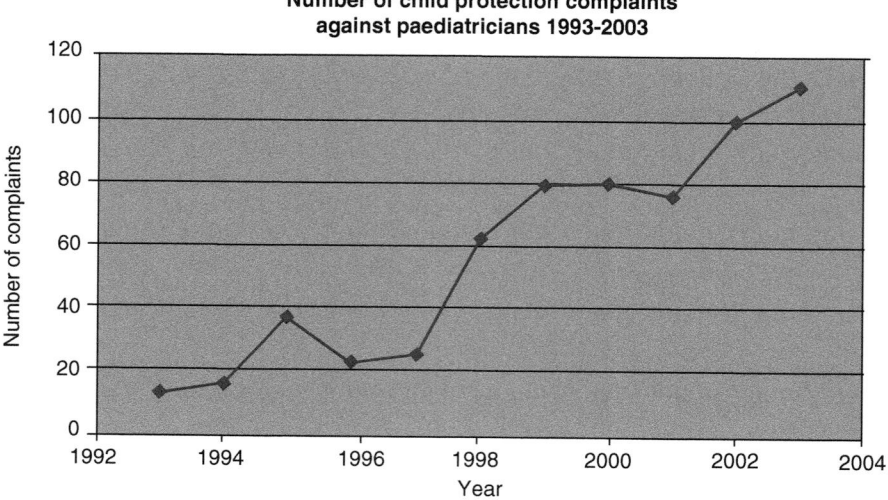

Number of child protection complaints against paediatricians 1993-2003

The RCPCH felt it could not be involved in individual cases but needed to represent the opinions of paediatricians. This lead to the GMC revising its guidance resulting in *Protecting Children and Young People: The Responsibilities of All Doctors*, produced following a 2-year working group chaired by senior family judge the Rt Hon Lord Justice Thorpe after hearing evidence from a range of child protection experts.

The College spent at least 10 years trying to improve support for paediatricians in the area of safeguarding. The aim was to make them competent in this core area of paediatrics so that they would feel confident to fulfil their vital role in this area. The latest manpower survey suggests that the tide may have turned and many trainees are keen to become involved.

Sexual Abuse

The case of the so-called Cleveland child abuse scandal emphasised the importance of correct interpretation of physical signs in suspected child sexual abuse. One of the main issues was the significance of the physical sign: reflex anal dilatation. Because of lack of evidence generally in the field of child sexual abuse in 1997, the Royal College of Physician's publication *Physical Signs of Sexual Abuse in Children* was published. This was based on the best evidence available at the time and revolutionised how evidence was given in court. This guidance was revised in 2008 with the publication by the RCPCH of the *The Physical Signs of Child Sexual Abuse: An Evidence-Based Review and Guidance to Best Practice*. The review focuses on evidence for the physical signs of child sexual abuse (CSA) in the following areas: female genitalia, male genitalia, anal signs, oral signs and sexually transmitted infections. A further edition was published in May 2015. Importantly this involved a fruitful collaboration with the American Academy of Pediatrics as well as the FLM of the RCPL. New chapters were included on genital bleeding and accidental genital injuries.

Network

The need to work collaboratively has never been greater and in 2010 the Department of Health and the RCPCH jointly commissioned a project, Child Protection Clinical Networks, in response to concerns about the contribution of health services in protecting children and young people from harm. This project has demonstrated the unique potential of managed clinical networks to protect children and support clinicians.

In the late 1990s, the RCPCH was made aware that the availability and the quality of safeguarding children training varied enormously across the UK and that the training was not mandatory. Under the leadership of the then President Prof Sir David Hall, the College had already begun to consider how to address this.

When Lord Laming's report into the tragic death of Victoria Climbié was published which highlighted, amongst other issues, the key roles and responsibilities of all paediatricians in safeguarding, the College had already set up a project group to urgently address the training needs of paediatricians. It was acknowledged that every paediatrician in training would have to take up recognised child protection courses as part of their training.

The RCPCH in collaboration with the NSPCC and the Department of Health set up a project (funded by the NSPCC, Department of Health and Johnson & Johnson Paediatric Institute) to develop the safeguarding training programmes for paediatricians – initially for trainees. The project was led by Dr Neela Shabde on behalf of the College in partnership with the Advanced Life Support Group (ALSG) and the NSPCC.

In January 2006, the first training package, *Safeguarding Children – Recognition and response in Child Protection*, was launched. This first-ever nationwide course was rolled out to all doctors in training in Paediatrics (ST1-4). The course was also considered appropriate for doctors training in emergency medicine and general practice.

In 2009, the same project group launched the next level of a training package: *Safeguarding Children – Child Protection in practice*. This is an e-learning modular course for ST4-7. A *Maintaining and Updating Competencies in Child Protection* a programme for consultants has also been produced.

Since then the College has developed a range of education and learning courses such as 'Child Protection: Examination to Court' which are heavily subscribed. Levels 4 and 5 safeguarding training for named and designated doctors, an e-learning programme on female genital mutilation and a legal report writing course are all now available. The CPSC and CPSIG have developed a SPIN module for child safeguarding for trainees and consultants who wish to develop a special interest in safeguarding.

Recognition and management of safeguarding issues is an integral part of every paediatricians work. The RCPCH has produced educational material and included safeguarding as a key part of training as well as continuing education.

Medicines for Children

18

David Hull, Imti Choonara, Helen Sammons, and Michael Beresford

The use of existing drugs and the development of new ones for use in children have been subject to many pressures, scientific, economic, social and political. In the period from 1970 to 1990, huge progress was made in the management of many serious illnesses in children utilising drugs which to a large extent were unlicensed for use in this age group. Indeed survival for children with leukaemia increased from 10 % in 1970 to almost 80 % by 1990, using drugs which had not been formally evaluated for use in children and for which no licensing or marketing authorisation had been sought or given. This is currently greater than 90 % because of most children now being part of a clinical trial as part of their treatment regimen in the UK.

The involvement of the BPA and then the college in this area began in 1991 with a letter to the then President, David Hull, from a group of parents with rare inherited metabolic disorders who were concerned that their children might not get the new medicines which were being developed for these conditions. Most of these products came direct from pharmaceutical companies and were largely untested and certainly unlicensed. The parents' concerns were fuelled by the changes in the structure of the NHS and the increasing effectiveness of the Medicines Licensing Authority. Hospital Trusts were beginning to have to carry their own burden of legal responsibility for the actions of their staff and unsurprisingly were not happy to see

D. Hull
Nottingham, UK

I. Choonara • H. Sammons (✉)
Derby, UK

M. Beresford
Liverpool, UK

© Springer International Publishing Switzerland 2017
A. Craft, K. Dodd (eds.), *From an Association to a Royal College*,
DOI 10.1007/978-3-319-43582-4_18

unlicensed products being prescribed and dispensed in their name on their premises. The task of the Licensing Authority was to protect the public. The Hospital Boards were acting in the general interests of the Trusts and even though this was for the general good it worked against the interests of children.

In response to these developments, the professions involved, paediatricians and paediatric pharmacists, with the support of the Department of Health, adopted a pragmatic approach involving the production of protocols and the development of networks. In the event these approaches were successful and the UK did not need to go down the US political route which led to their Orphan Drug Legislation.

In 1992, a report appeared suggesting that Vitamin K, which was widely used across the UK to prevent haemorrhagic disease of the newborn, might be associated with an increased risk of childhood cancer. This attracted a great deal of media attention. Vitamin K, IM had been on the market for many years, long before licensing had been established. Some paediatricians, who had been concerned about untoward incidents with the IM injections, had already moved to giving it orally on the grounds that vitamins can be considered as foods and therefore might avoid any drug regulatory issues. There was no oral product so the liquid injection was given by mouth for which it had no licence and was therefore considered to be 'off label'.

Some midwives and health visitors, on learning this, took legal advice through their professional organisations and on the basis of this refused to give it. They acted as they saw it in the interests of their professional standards. Such high standards normally bring significant benefit but in this instance put babies at a serious disadvantage. This problem could clearly not be resolved with protocols and networks.

About that time the CMO in Scotland had noted that the teaching hospitals in that country were issuing guidelines on the administration of medicines to children but that they often differed between the hospitals and could be out of date. He wrote to the BPA suggesting that the production of a paediatric formulary was a task for the BPA. He indicated there might be some funds available for this. It was when he met his colleagues in England that the President of the BPA received a carefully worded letter. The Department of Health advised ministers who were the Licensing Authority, and they could not be seen to be supporting an endeavour which might recommend the use of unlicensed medicines. Given the positions of the authorities, it was clear that those who had a duty of care for sick children were heading for trouble. Political action was possible but even if it were able to address the issues, it would take time. The BPA decided to act. They met with the Association of the British Pharmaceutical Industry (ABPI) and the Neonatal and Paediatric Pharmacists Group (NPPG). They issued a joint statement on the issues as they saw them and indicated areas where they wished to see progress (*Licensing Medicines for Children, 1996*).

These issues included the need to consider developmental biology and possible age bands where advice might be different. There was a need for clinical appraisal of drugs and any known differences in pharmacokinetics. In order to ensure safety, it would be necessary to set up a serious side effect surveillance system for unlicensed medications. Finally, it would be necessary to provide information available and accessible to all. All of these areas were subsequently addressed in a variety of ways.

Information was one area that paediatricians and pharmacists could do something about, and producing guidance on medicines suitable for children would address many of these unmet needs. The production of a formulary was the first and important step. The publication of *Medicines for Children* (MfC) was funded by a generous grant from the Nuffield Foundation and was a huge step forward.

The primary purpose was to collect together best practice to ensure children were treated as well as possible. The guidance was as evidence based as it could be. Many paediatricians and paediatric pharmacists from across the UK gave freely of their time to complete this huge exercise. The book emphasised generic names, and it stuck to an agreed age banding structure across all sections irrespective of what any licensing recommendations might say. The licensing status of the drug was emphasised as most clinicians were at that time unaware that many drugs they were using were unlicensed for children. It excluded all of the detail on the product information leaflets which did not apply to children. The hope that bringing to the attention the fact that their drugs were being used unlicensed for children might provoke manufacturers into making public any information they had on the drug's use in children and perhaps even apply for a licence. Unfortunately, this aspiration was not realised and most drugs remain unlicensed.

MfC contained protocols of care under the imprimatur of the RCPCH and the NPPG. It was hoped that this would go some way to reassure Trusts that those who administered unlicensed and off-label medications to children were acting reasonably and that this would deter any legal action. There is no doubt that MfC was extremely well received by paediatricians, and it went through three editions. But one of the problems was accessibility. MfC had to be bought and many Trusts would only purchase a limited number. At the same time, every junior and senior doctor was given a free copy of the British National Formulary every 6 months. This was primarily an adult-focussed production and did not contain the professional consensus advice as in MfC. Indeed the advice about prescribing for children was often confusing. By this stage the RCPCH had been formed, and they used their growing political influence to persuade the Department of Health to fund the production of a separate British National Formulary for Children (BNF-C). Dr George Rylance who had been a senior editor of MfC took on the task of preparing a BNF-C. There was much negotiation necessary as the BNF was a joint publication of the British Medical Association and the Royal Pharmaceutical Society. The BNF was bought by the Department of Health and distributed to all practising doctors in the NHS so a special arrangement had to be made for those working primarily with children. The first edition of BNF-C appeared in September 2005 and has become the standard source of information on prescribing medicines for children in the UK. It has also been adapted for use in countries including India, Italy and New Zealand.

But this was not the end of the matter. MfC was largely based on consensus as so little investigation had been undertaken on most drugs used in children. There was still a real feeling that for the future the needs of children must be considered when new drugs were in the development phase, and if possible the necessary data should be obtained to apply for retrospective licensing for the many commonly used drugs.

In 2004 the RCPCH produced a report entitled *Safer and Better Medicines for Children*. Following this and the landmark papers in the BMJ and Arch Dis Child Fetal and Neonatal Edition lobbying by the RCPCH along with that from other EU member states culminated in the European Union 'Paediatric Regulation' in 2007. This has meant that all new medicines, appropriate for use in children, must be researched in this population. *Paediatric-use marketing authorisation (PUMA)* aims to stimulate research in unlicensed and off-label medicines. Companies benefit from 10 years of data protection as a reward for the development of a new indication in children or formulations appropriate for children of all ages. This legislation however has failed to produce good results, with only one medication (buccal midazolam) being approved so far.

Training in Paediatric Clinical Pharmacology

In August 2000, the RCPCH initiated a meeting on training in paediatric clinical pharmacology; alongside members of the RCPCH were individuals from the Royal College of Physicians with an interest in training in adult clinical pharmacology and therapeutics. It was agreed that the RCPCH should play a key role in the training of paediatric clinical pharmacology. Also that such individuals should be paediatricians and that alongside a curriculum and training programme, the long-term aim should be to establish a College Specialist Advisory Committee (CSAC). The working group invited representation from the pharmaceutical industry, as they were having involvement in training in adult clinical pharmacology. Over the next 2 years, a training programme was developed.

In 2003, the Specialist Training Authority (STA) approved paediatric clinical pharmacology as a sub-speciality of paediatrics. In 2003, a training post in paediatric clinical pharmacology was established in Derby. Individuals were also receiving training in London and Aberdeen, and in 2004, the first college, CSAC of Paediatric Clinical Pharmacology, was established. Unfortunately, it was not possible to establish formal training programmes in either London or Aberdeen as they did not have a paediatric clinical pharmacologist in post.

In 2006, Dr Helen Sammons completed her training and was awarded a CCT in Paediatric Clinical Pharmacology (the first accredited individual in the sub-speciality in the UK). Subsequently, several other individuals have completed their training and have taken up posts throughout the UK. Paediatric clinical pharmacologists are currently in posts in Derby and Liverpool.

Developing an Infrastructure for Clinical Trials of Medicines in Children in the UK

This was undertaken on behalf of the Medical Research Council, the Department of Health and the Association of the British Pharmaceutical Industry. The report emphasised that children were being denied the fundamental right of safe and effective medicines. This very unsatisfactory state of affairs had been recognised in the USA, and legislation had put in place real incentives for the pharmaceutical industry to include children in the development of new drugs. The USA had set up a network of paediatric pharmacology centres in which the necessary studies could be undertaken. The RCPCH report called for a similar network to be set up in the UK. The Department of Health decided against this but instead set up an NIHR Medicine for Children Research Network to encourage centres to enter children into clinical trials with the aim of eventually getting the data to ensure that more drugs are licensed for use in children. This was created in 2005 and included the MCRN Coordinating Centre in Liverpool, UK, 6 Local Research Networks (LRNs) across England, 12 Clinical Studies Groups (CSGs) covering most paediatric specialty areas, Clinical Trial Units (CTUs) and a Neonatal Network. In 2013, this was merged within the NIHR Clinical Research Network (CRN) and a Children's stream was created. This brought together MCRN and the Paediatric (non-medicines) Specialty Group to cover all children's research. This continues to be supported by college members and has considerable liaison with college committees to drive research forward. Further work to enable existing drugs to be retrospectively licensed for children though the European Union has funded some work through the FP7 projects. The college also provides suggestions for topics to the MRC and other national funders, surrounding children's medicines.

Medicines for Children: Safe and Reliable Advice for Parents and MEDS IQ

This is a joint project between the RCPCH, the Neonatal and Paediatric Pharmacists Group (NPPG) and the national children's charity WellChild (http://www.medicinesforchildren.org.uk/). The work was started in 2006 with a project team from the above groups and is now progressing under the guidance of the Joint RCPCH/ NPPG Medicines Committee. The aims of this work were to make information in an easily understood form available for parents and children themselves. Simple advice on how to give the drug and what to do if a dose was missed or the child vomited was included and has proven very useful.

This project is now in its tenth year and continues to provide appropriate and accurate information about medicine dosages, side effects and general advice to those giving medicines to children and young people in their care. A medical text writer works with the WellChild parent/carer's group to ensure the text is written to an appropriate reading age and style, and leaflets have received information standard accreditation. The website was launched in 2009 and has recently been revamped to make it more user-friendly. It now contains just under 200 leaflets and 7 videos freely available to all. The leaflets are referenced for individual medicines in the most recent edition of the BNF-C, and information is given in the personal child health record (red book).

The MEDS IQ project (http://www.medsiq.org/) was launched in 2015 by the college. Medication errors are a significant but preventable cause of harm to children and young people. MEDS IQ aims to bring together tools and improvement projects that have been developed to address this problem. The vision is that child health professionals will be able to use this resource to support their own improvement work and learn from the experiences of others. At the same time, MEDS IQ is bringing together organisations across the UK and beyond to ensure that medication safety remains a priority for paediatric research and practice.

The RCPCH's continued administrative and financial support of these projects, along with that from the other project partners, has been essential in the success of them.

International

Peter B. Sullivan and Bhanu Williams

There had been a long history of linkages between paediatric units in Britain and those in the developing world. There were, for instance, linkages between paediatric units in London, Newcastle, Liverpool and Exeter with units overseas from the early 1950s. Heinz Fellowships were inaugurated in 1961 to assist British paediatricians to make short visits to developing countries and overseas paediatricians to attend the annual meeting of the British Paediatric Association (BPA) and to visit academic paediatric centres. By 1964 these links were becoming so common that the BPA Council appointed an Overseas Committee to oversee the arrangement of the programmes of Heinz Fellows and their supervisors. Their remit was also to review the arrangements for postgraduate education of overseas students in Britain, as well as the training of British graduates in tropical paediatrics. The booklet 'Paediatric training in the United Kingdom' (1968) ran to four editions and provided information about education in paediatrics for overseas postgraduates.

The Tropical Paediatric Group was formed in the early 1970s by British paediatricians who had worked in the developing world. It became one of the first British Paediatric Association specialist groups. Tropical child health continued to be a focus of interest of the BPA reflecting the long tradition of significant contributions made to this discipline by several illustrious British paediatricians. Cicely Williams, for instance, had started maternal and child health clinics in the Gold Coast (now Ghana) in the 1930s. Derek Jelliffe was appointed to the first UNICEF chair of

P.B. Sullivan
Oxford, UK

B. Williams (✉)
London, UK

© Springer International Publishing Switzerland 2017
A. Craft, K. Dodd (eds.), *From an Association to a Royal College*,
DOI 10.1007/978-3-319-43582-4_19

paediatrics and child health at Makerere College, Uganda, where he founded the first journal of tropical paediatrics. In 1985, as result of growing membership and a feeling that perhaps the name of the Group was too limiting, the International Child Health Group (ICHG) emerged out of the Tropical Paediatric Group. The ICHG continues to be a very active specialty group of the Royal College of Paediatrics and Child Health.

The further development of the international dimension in the newly formed Royal College of Paediatrics and Child Health was catalysed by one of the most tragic incidents in the history of the college. David Baum, President of the College, died of a heart attack on 5 September 1999 whilst cycling from Buckingham Palace to Sandringham to raise funds for the college's work in Kosovo and Gaza. David Baum had created and chaired an International Task Force on Children affected by War and Absolute Poverty from 1997 with the aim of improving care of children in the most disadvantaged areas of the world by promoting education and training of paediatricians. It was decided the college would both commemorate David and continue his work through creation of an Officer for International Affairs, the David Baum Fellow, and the establishment of the David Baum International Foundation (DBIF). The Foundation was officially launched on 30 January 2001 at a very happy occasion in Hallam Street attended by many of David's family. The blueprint for the role of the Officer for International Affairs had, in fact, already been drawn up by Tim Chambers in his strategy paper on International Relations for the college in June 1999.

It was against the background of David Baum's active interest in the welfare of children caught up in warfare, and particularly in the Balkans conflict, that the college was asked if it would be willing to help in advising on a training and education programme for the Department of Paediatrics and Neonatology in Pristina, Kosovo. Dr Doug Johnston took this forward and worked indefatigably to improve child health services in Kosovo and was instrumental in the development of a curriculum for postgraduate paediatric training in that country. In May 2000 the new President, David Hall, led a delegation to Pristina to provide the first external lectures for Kosovan paediatricians following the withdrawal of the Serbian troops.

The college's work in Gaza followed an approach to RCPCH by Lady Patience Moberley of Medical Aid for Palestine (MAP) to offer a teaching programme in Gaza for paediatricians in 1998. A workshop in Gaza followed and was attended by David Baum, Alan Craft, Tom Lissauer, the Minister of Health and MAP.

The British government, through the Department for International Development, helped support this initiative. The following year, Tony Waterston was appointed to lead the Gaza project. Considerable logistical and political difficulties thwarted progress, but by 2005, a pilot teaching programme in the West Bank was underway. Within 2 years of this, 'Juzoor' A Palestinian NGO for health and social development and Al-Quds Medical School, key partners in the West Bank, took on local organisation and initiated a Diploma in Palestinian Child Health.

At the millennium, one in ten members and Fellows of the College practised paediatrics abroad, and a questionnaire survey revealed that they would like to see a more structured way through which to interact with the college. Specifically, more input for training of young paediatricians and Fellowships for clinical science research training were requested. It was clear from the survey that there was also a considerable demand for RCPCH-endorsed clinical practice guidelines and standards of clinical care for children. The demand for college postgraduate examinations not only remained popular but increased in demand in a number of predominately Commonwealth countries. Following this survey, in 2001, the Council endorsed the setting up of an Overseas Linkage Programme. The objectives of this programme were to encourage partnership between the college and overseas colleagues and provide a 'two-way street' for the exchange of ideas and information. Resources were limited so projects needed to be very focussed and have a good chance of producing long-term gains for the overseas partner. The lack of a specific budget for international affairs was proving to be a significant handicap, and, following a motion proposed by the ICHG in 2001, college members voted at the AGM for an additional levy of 2 % to be added onto the membership subscriptions to fund development of overseas activity. This together with funds from DBIF created the opportunity to establish some of these Overseas Linkages.

One example of such a linkage was with the Kilimanjaro Christian Medical Centre (KCMC) in Tanzania. The first in a series of planned training visits took place in April 2003 and provided not only an opportunity to deliver on-site training but also to undertake a detailed needs assessment to ensure that future input was targeted on the training needs of the institution. Miss Kokila Lakhoo, a paediatric surgeon, Georgina Hall and Richard Coward had made further visits, and in addition to advice on training and reorganising the paediatric unit, infrastructure was also provided by way of medical books and slide projectors as part of the project. Work in Tanzania was extended (2004–2006) to Muhimbili Hospital in Dar es Salaam with delivery of two medical education training courses and an evidence-based medicine course. Further work in East Africa was supported by DBIF with the ETAT-Plus course, a partnership project which provides training in Emergency Triage Assessment and Treatment run by Mike English and colleagues in Nairobi from 2005.

The first ever visits by college officers to accredit overseas units for postgraduate paediatric training for UK trainees were made in 2002 at the KEMRI-Kilifi research unit in Kenya and at Queen Elizabeth Hospital, Blantyre, Malawi. These visits were undertaken at the invitation of the Wellcome Trust, and both units were awarded college certification for their excellent postgraduate paediatric training programmes.

Two events in 2003 were notable; one was the joint venture between the college and the Rhodes Trust in hosting a meeting at Magdalen College, Oxford, entitled 'Paediatric Education for Capacity Building in Developing Countries', aimed to (i) provide an overview of the health of children in the developing world, (ii) outline a programme of skill transfer initiatives designed to train a network of health workers who will provide a focus for efforts to tackle the major health problems confronting children in Southern Africa and (iii) bring together the academic, governmental and non-governmental agencies with an interest in developing and contributing to the college's international programmes. Paediatricians from Africa and Southeast Asia were invited to the meeting which was chaired by the college's patron, Her Royal Highness the Princess Royal, who had consistently supported the college's international activities.

Following the second Gulf War Iraq had been under the rule of Saddam Hussein for many years and as a result of this and international sanctions, Iraqi doctors were effectively cut off from the rest of the world. The college lost no time in engaging with Iraqi paediatricians following the change in regime and in December 2004 ran the first of a series of training courses in Amman, Jordan. This engagement was supported by the Jordanian Paediatric Society, the British Council, the British Ambassador to Jordan, Mr Christopher Prentice and His Royal Highness Prince El Hassan bin Talal of the Hashemite Kingdom of Jordan. When the security situation improved from 2009, further courses were run in Iraq itself in partnership with the Ministry of Health in Kurdistan and Hawler Medical University, Erbil.

The International Paediatric Training Scheme (IPTS) operated for several years under the auspices of the college. The scheme allowed suitably qualified paediatricians to obtain limited registration with the GMC to practise and train in the UK. Another scheme was the RCPCH/VSO Fellowship scheme which has offered trainees with their MRCPCH a 12-month opportunity to share their skills in a developing country supported in their work by one or two senior doctors, who act as supervisors. This joint venture has supported placements in Malawi, Namibia, the Gambia and Uganda and other countries, and in some cases this has been recognised as part of their formal training.

The college was also active in South Asia with Memoranda of Understanding with both the Indian Academy of Pediatrics and the Pakistan Paediatric Association. Close links were formed with the College of Physicians and Surgeons in Bangladesh following a visit by the President in 2002 and by the David Baum Fellow in 2005. From 2006, a programme called 'Training in Evidence-Based Medicine in India' was funded by the David Baum International Foundation and aimed to provide Indian paediatricians with the skills needed to use research evidence appropriately and integrate it with their clinical practice. These courses have taken place in Bangalore, Chandigarh and Delhi. It is expected that new centres will take on the courses and eventually that the Indian Academy of Pediatrics will take over running courses across India. RCPCH continues to raise standards for paediatricians overseas through examinations held in a wide range of low- and middle-income countries and regions around the world.

Opportunities for overseas paediatricians to visit the UK to obtain experience in paediatrics are afforded by a number of international scholarships administered by the college. These include the Donald Court and Heinz Fellowships and the Douglas Hubble Travel Bursary. An additional bursary, the Ashok Nathwani Fellowship, was created in 2002 in memory of one of the College Fellows who was very active in international affairs and who was tragically killed in an Indian Earthquake in January 2001. The college also donated 100,000 rupees to the children's hospital in Ahmedabad as a bequest in Dr Nathwani's memory.

In 2007, Steven Greene took over from Peter Sullivan as David Baum Fellow, and, as the range and extent of international activities had expanded so rapidly from the millennium, he was joined by three new Overseas Directors with specific geographical remits. These were Ezzedin Gouta (Middle East), Mike Webb (India) and, for Africa, Steve Allen who went on in 2011 to become the third David Baum Fellow. In 2016, RCPCH conducted a second membership survey on our international work. One hundred percent of respondents supported the principle of RCPCH engagement in global health. Sixty-six percent advocated for that engagement to grow.

In 2015 Bhanu Williams became the fourth David Baum Fellow. From 2015, a new RCPCH global strategy was endorsed by the college and put into operation. The strategy aims to consolidate, organise and enhance the impact of the extensive range of RCPCH and members' international interests and activities. The overarching strategic focus is on ensuring the RCPCH international (now 'RCPCH Global') activities all contribute to building the capacity of health workers in low-income (and where relevant middle-income) countries. The strategy is based on the premise that what the RCPCH offers more than anything else is one of the greatest concentrations of paediatric knowledge and skills in the world. We believe that it is by transferring those skills, by situating ourselves and working alongside doctors, nurses, midwives, interns and others in resource-poor hospitals and health facilities, that we have the greatest and most sustained impact on the quality of health care, and the strengthening of health systems in countries undergoing development.

Under the circumstances of the Millennium Development Goals and the newly launched Sustainable Development Goals, RCPCH's global health work has a central focus on improving global maternal, newborn and child health outcomes. Much of this will be achieved through strengthening clinical care through evidence-based capacity building, training and education. But we remain committed to the wider remit of child health – to ensuring action on chronic conditions, nutrition and obesity, adolescent sexual and mental health. We aim further to build the presence and reputation of the Royal College of Paediatrics and Child Health as a leading voice and actor in global health by building a coherent body of global health work, funded by a range of donors, maximising the potential of the RCPCH members, staff and partners.

As of February 2016, RCPCH holds a total of £1.25 million in grants for global child health capacity building work. Donors include DFID through the Tropical Health Education Trust (THET), Jersey Overseas Aid (JOA) and UNICEF. Much of our recent work has been centred on strengthening emergency facility-based care for critically unwell children through the WHO validated Emergency Triage Assessment and Treatment programme. Working in partnership with local paediatricians and Ministries of Health, RCPCH has supported training and mentoring clinicians in multiple sites in East Africa and Myanmar.

Our model of partnership is based on long-term volunteering, ensuring a high level of value for money in programme funding terms. But it is also based on mutual learning – the increasingly compelling evidence that for every volunteer taking time out of the NHS to work with colleagues in low-income countries and clinics, the British health system receives back clinicians with sharpened clinical acumen, improved leadership and management skills and a renewed commitment to child health.

Since 2012 the RCPCH Global Links programme has placed over 60 trainees, consultants and retired consultants in 28 district and tertiary level hospitals in Kenya, Uganda, Sierra Leone, Ghana and Myanmar. Volunteers work alongside local healthcare staff to role-model good clinical practice, offer much needed in-service continuing medical education and train in the use of clinical audit and quality improvement methodologies.

RCPCH has established a strong presence in East Africa, building emergency care skills for children in hospitals in Kenya, Uganda and Rwanda. Our regional partnerships – with government, paediatric associations, medical schools and university departments – provide the basis on which to extend a programme model with proven capacity to drive down infant and child deaths, for example, expanding our reach to work with health centres in Kibera – one of the world's largest slum settlements.

We have expanded our work in West Africa – initially through a 'Global Links' volunteer programme in Sierra Leone. Following the 2014 Ebola outbreak in that country, we are developing a programme of work, in consultation with government and partners, to support reconstruction of the health sector. This new programme aims to harness the collective potential of multiple Medical Royal Colleges, to build and streamline the UK's overarching model of global health partnership.

In 2015 we launched a new project funded by UKAid and the Tropical Health Education Trust (THET), working with the Paediatric Society of Palestine, to train local health providers in multidisciplinary approaches to children with disabilities. RCPCH has also worked with Juzoor for Health and Development to develop a unique Diploma in Child Health delivered in Palestine and subsequently developed into a Masters in Child Health (MACH) with Al-Quds University.

Within the UK, RCPCH and ICHG members have developed a set of global child health competencies for all UK-based clinicians which were published in the Lancet in 2014 – many of which will be included in the new RCPCH curriculum. Since 2012, RCPCH has delivered a Child Health in Low Resource Settings course to train UK clinicians to work abroad. We plan to develop a training track to develop future leaders in global child health. We continue to advocate for the most vulnerable children globally through briefings and representation in UK parliament, partnership discussions with Ministries of Health and publications in national newspapers and leading medical journals, most recently in a 2015 Lancet Comment on the Sustainable Development Goals.

From its earliest origins, the RCPCH has been a leading voice in defending and promoting the health of infants, children and young people in the UK and internationally. Over time, we have seen that health has become global – that child health too has become a global issue and that caring for children is an overriding imperative, regardless of geography. As we go forward, we aim to build the RCPCH's ability to understand, through research, the issues affecting child health at a global level, to take action on those issues where we have the skills and to speak out to those with the power to change things where we do not.

Nursing

20

Sue Burr and Fiona Smith

Close working relationships had been established with children's nurses in the time of the BPA. It was commonplace in the 1980s and 1990s for children to be nursed on adult wards and by generally trained nurses rather than those with children's training, and the BPA worked hard to rectify this. A joint approach through working parties and the several reports of the group 'Caring for Children in the Health Service' helped to achieve change, but the establishment of the RCPCH brought greater influence (e.g. the establishment of a minister for children, children's commissioners and a national service framework for children).

Sue Burr and Fiona Smith were our key links with the RCN through this period and have played important roles in improving the nursing care of sick children.

Reflections of Nursing, Sue Burr and Fiona Smith (RCN Advisers in Paediatric Nursing, 1984–2002 and 2001–Present)

The Royal College of Nursing had a long history of representation on committees and working groups of other professional and governmental organisations and regularly responded to such organisation's documents around issues relating to children and young people's nursing. Prior to the 1980s, the RCN had within its formal structures groups of members termed 'associations' or 'societies' and for smaller groups 'forums' for members with interests or qualifications in areas such as education, cancer, management and mental health. However those members of RCN who had the registered sick children's nurse (RSCN) qualification and were working with children had no formal structure of support or representation. It was not unusual

S. Burr
Dorset, UK

F. Smith (✉)
London, UK

© Springer International Publishing Switzerland 2017
A. Craft, K. Dodd (eds.), *From an Association to a Royal College*,
DOI 10.1007/978-3-319-43582-4_20

for the RCN to nominate a member to an outside body relating to children who did not have the RSCN qualification.

The RCN's Institute of Education had a worldwide reputation for post-registration training courses with many nurses attending from overseas, especially from former commonwealth countries. In spite of many of these countries having a huge health problem with children, the RCN did not provide courses concerned with the nursing of children.

In 1984, following lobbying from members of the RCN, Sue Burr, a member of staff with an RSCN qualification, was appointed with the title of Adviser in Paediatric Nursing. One of the Adviser's specific tasks was to establish a society of paediatric nursing and smaller forums for the speciality groups. The Paediatric Oncology Nurses Forum was the first to be established in June 1984. This appointment met with some opposition which was not dissimilar to the attitude of some of the ancient medical royal colleges in the transition from BPA to RCPCH. It was perhaps not surprising that the Nurse Adviser received excellent support from the BPA, and likewise the RCN provided support to the BPA in the establishment of the RCPCH. The Paediatric Nurse Adviser along with the Chairman of the society or relevant forum assumed responsibility for nominating appropriate representatives on outside bodies and responding to requests for advice. Since 1984 only those who are registered children's nurses can fulfil this role.

In 1984, few registered children's nurses were employed in small children's units. The appointment by the RCN of a Paediatric Nurse Adviser gave both paediatricians and nurses working in these units a named person with whom they could share their concerns, seek advice or be put in touch with an appropriate expert. In addition they were alerted to relevant policies and guidance issued by governmental, voluntary and professional bodies. This enabled paediatricians to be more supportive to the nursing staff and assisted them in being more proactive in working with management.

In addition, post-registration courses, and then a degree in child health nursing, were developed by the RCN. The RCN Journal of Paediatric Nursing (now Nursing Children and Young People) was the first UK journal concerned solely with the nursing of children and young people, and the BPA/RCPCH explicitly welcomed these important developments.

The support of the BPA/RCPCH has been very important to the Paediatric Nurse Adviser. The post is seen as a very busy and lonely post in an organisation whose main priorities lie with adult health and illness. Sue Burr was the first nurse to be elected as an honorary member of the BPA, and she then became a Founding Fellow of the RCPCH. This acknowledgment by an outside body greatly enhanced the struggle for proper recognition of paediatric nursing within the family of nursing. The BPA/RCPCH provided support for the retention of the child branch pre-registration programmes and relevant specialist paediatric and neonatal education programmes.

More recently the RCN have reciprocated with the award of an Hon. FRCN to four former officers of the RCPCH, Patricia Hamilton in 2009, Alan Craft in 2013, Sheila Shribman in 2014 and Hilary Cass in 2016.

In addition to the formal mechanisms for sharing expertise with enquiries from paediatricians and the College, the Nursing Adviser has been able to provide solid facts and supporting evidence to strengthen the production of important policies and documents. Paediatricians and children's nurses who wanted to develop a specific aspect of a service, e.g. community nursing for sick and disabled children, have been able to work together under the strength of the two organisations for the benefits of children.

Since the advent of the paediatric nurse adviser (now the Adviser in Children and Young People's Nursing), there has been a considerable change in the way that advice about children's nursing is sought.

Prior to the founding of the RCPCH, all documents that might have an impact on children were sent to the medical royal colleges and the RCN, but not the BPA. The paediatric nurse adviser would alert the Honorary Secretary of the BPA of such documents, and he could request a copy for the BPA to comment separately. When the BPA became a college, it automatically received such documents. When the relevance of the document to children was not obvious from the title, e.g. Accident and Emergency Nursing, the RCPCH would alert the Paediatric Adviser at the RCN.

The growing recognition of the nursing needs of children and the necessity to work across organisations to influence government led to the formation of an organisation in 1985: Caring for Children in the Health Service. This was an organisation under the umbrella of the RCN and BPA with the National Association for the Welfare of Children in Hospital (NAWCH) and the National Association of Health Authorities and Trusts (NAHAT). They first met to discuss concerns about the lack of research relating to the health care of children, and they agreed to seek monies to undertake specific pieces of research to highlight the needs of children in the NHS. It was an unusual organisation which had no constitution, no fees and no officers other than the chair Lady Jean Lovell-Davies. The BPA published the reports, the RCN organised press conferences and NAWCH provided the chair. The first piece of research entitled 'Where are the Children' published in 1987 highlighted the fact that, years after the Platt report in 1959, many children were still being cared for in adult wards with little or no paediatric input and no qualified paediatric nurses (now known as children's nurses). Six further pieces of work related to children's health were completed:

- *Where are the children?* An Examination of Regional Statistics for Children in Hospital and the Implications regarding Agreed Standards of Care, 1987
- *Hidden children*, 1998
- *Parents staying overnight with their children in hospital*, 1998.
- *Just for the day*: Children admitted to hospital for day treatment, 1991
- *Bridging the gaps*: An exploratory study of the interfaces between primary and specialist care for children within the health services, 1993
- *Youth matters*: Evidence-based best practice for the care of young people in hospital, 1998.

As a result of these reports, children were undoubtedly moved up the political agenda. After the first report, a meeting was requested with the Secretary of State and surprisingly was granted, probably on the grounds that it was most unusual at that time to have different organisations working together on behalf of children. There is little doubt that the authority of each of these organisations was enhanced by the process.

Since 1985 the number of joint publications between the RCN and the BPA/RCPCH has increased considerably, and the joint statements, joint working groups, conferences, study days, learning resources, standards, recommendations and a united front have all helped to strengthen services for children and young people.

The annual meeting of the RCPCH is now badged as joint between RCPCH and RCN, and there is increasing nursing input.

Archives of Disease in Childhood (ADC)

21

Mark Beattie and Bernard Valman

Revelations of an insider at the Archives of Disease in Childhood, Bernard Valman, Editor ADC 1992 – 1994 and Commissioning Editor 1994–1999 updated by the Mark Beattie, Editor 2012 -

How was a journal 'fit for wrapping fish and chips' [1] transformed into an international organisation with more than 2000 papers submitted, papers posted online soon after they have been accepted, a wide variety of review articles published for the general reader, more than three million downloads per year and a circulation of many thousands (print) with extensive international access through consortia and institutional subscriptions?

ADC was founded by the British Medical Association (BMA) as the first house specialist journal in 1926. In Britain there were about 50 physicians with a special interest in diseases of children and a handful who worked exclusively with children. The editor of the BMJ, Sir Dawson Williams wrote 'Some of the medical men whose work lies mainly among children had suggested that the BMA should publish a new journal' [2]. Williams had been a paediatrician before becoming a full-time journalist, and this may have influenced his decision to support this risky proposal. The British Journal of Children's Diseases had been published from 1904 and was a competitor for the small number of subscriptions. At the first meeting of the Archives' editorial committee, the present title was adopted, and Hugh Thursfield and Reginald Miller were appointed the first joint editors [3]. Sir Thomas Barlow stated in his introduction to the first edition that the reasons for the publication were that conclusions scattered through various publications should be available, there should be

Part of this material is republished with permission from Valman B. Revelations of an Insider: ADC 1926–2006. Arch Dis Child 2006; 91: 962–966

M. Beattie (✉)
Southampton, UK

B. Valman
London, UK

© Springer International Publishing Switzerland 2017
A. Craft, K. Dodd (eds.), *From an Association to a Royal College*,
DOI 10.1007/978-3-319-43582-4_21

opportunities for research to be published and criticised and adoption of research into practice should be promoted [4]. The journal has remained true to this mission even if the terminology has changed – publishing original research to impact on practice, review articles on topical issues, editorials to highlight specific content and review articles and editorials and high quality content accredited for professional development. Getting research into practice through quality improvement and implementation of science remains at the centre of the journal's mission [5].

Associate Editors

When I (Bernard Valman) was appointed twin editor with Roy Meadow in 1982, we were faced with an increasing number of submitted articles, the developing specialties in paediatrics and a long delay before publication. Editors of journals for the general reader such as the BMJ and the Archives were worried about the long-term future because authors at the cutting edge of their specialties were sending their best papers to the organ specialty journals, and there was a danger that the general journals would receive only the rejects. I wrote to Jerold Lucey, the editor of the American Academy of Pediatrics journal *Pediatrics*, and he invited me to meet all the American editors of paediatric journals at the annual meeting of the association in San Francisco. I outlined the problems and asked for their opinions about the appointment of associate editors. They all objected because they said that associate editors would favour their own specialty and produce an imbalance of papers for the general reader. Despite this advice we appointed Malcolm Chiswick as the first associate editor for foetal and neonatal medicine in 1995, and his effectiveness was followed by the appointment of associate editors in other specialties. The *Journal of Pediatrics* and most of the other international paediatric journals quickly followed this pattern. The long waiting time for publication was resolved by reducing the acceptance rate temporarily until more pages became available and the major emerging specialities were given associate editors. These specialist papers were balanced by a considerable increase in the popular review articles for the general reader, which also kept the specialists up to date with developments outside their fields.

There are now 24 editions published each year including the main or 'blue' journal, Fetal and Neonatal Edition and Education and Practice. The journal has an editor-in-chief, 3 edition editors, a commissioning editor, 5 deputy editors, a senior editor, 19 associate editors, 10 section editors for Education and Practice, a statistical editor and a team of statistical advisors. There is also a global health editor and editors for Archimedes (evidence-based reviews), images and the social media. Michael Healy was the first statistical advisor and, when he retired from the chair at the London School of Tropical Medicine and Hygiene, he attended all the fortnightly selection meetings so that all papers for publication were assessed by him and helpful suggestions given to authors. Tim Cole now leads the team of statistical editors with all complex submissions which include significant statistical content being reviewed by his team.

The journal editorial process runs paperlight and mostly by conference call – this has enabled the editorial team (national and international) to get involved in the decision making 'hanging committee' where the best submissions are selected for publications based on their content, quality and relevance to the readership. The editorial team has become more international with editors from Europe, the USA and Australia.

The journal, co-owned by the RCPCH and BMJ, benefits considerably form the much expanded publishing team with the technical editor and assistant being replaced by a publisher, managing editor, editorial assistant and production editor supported by staff with expertise in social media, marketing, plagiarism, ethics and the press.

Technology

In 1983, the journal changed from 'hot metal type' made by Linotype setters, and composed in trays, to computer setting. We no longer corrected long strips of galley proofs that had been produced by pressing a sheet of paper against the inked type, using the technique employed by Caxton. We still need to check proofs sent to us by email for electronic correction. The importance of interesting, well set-out, accurate, easy to work through and relevant information has not changed.

Since 2002 all papers have been submitted and refereed by email. A research paper may travel thousands of miles in up to 10 journeys before acceptance, with a median time to a first decision of 36 days. It may be placed on the website to be seen by readers within weeks of acceptance. There are an increasing number of hits at the website with the highest number from the USA and the second from the UK. In 2015 there were 10,000,000 website page impressions and 3,000,000 downloads (plus 750,000 for the Fetal and Neonatal Edition and 160,000 for Education and Practice). We can tell who reads what and where and what our most popular papers are – practical papers that help doctors make better decisions do the best – previously called 'personal practice' and now called things like 'recent advances', 'investigation and management' and 'best practice'.

Podcasts were launched in 2008 and are now weekly. *Online First* was introduced in 2010 and provides the *EPUB* of the paper ahead of the print edition. The paper is edited, typeset and approved by the author so that it can be cited. The journal has Twitter and Facebook accounts for the different editions, regular email alerts, hot topic alerts and most recently a Twitter journal club.

Finance

In 1997, the BMA and the BPA became equal partners sharing the profits or losses with up to 800 free copies given to BPA members. In 1980 the BPA twice demanded the yearly subscription from members; to avoid bankruptcy, the national inflation rate was 27%. Following a new contract in 1981, the journal produced high profits for the BMA and BPA, who kept them in a reserve fund that was later used to provide a substantial part of the cost of the first college building in Hallam Street. These profits encouraged the finance committee to increase the number of pages printed each year from 992 quarto to 1540 A4 by 1992. The majority of the extra pages were used for review articles to keep the journal attractive to the general reader. The journal is now jointly owned by the Royal College of Paediatrics and Child Health (formed from the BPA in 1996) and the British Medical Journals established as a separate company from the BMA in the early 2000s. There are now 24 editions published each year – 2124 pages. The journal's finances remain in healthy positive balance.

Content

In the early years, there were long descriptions of disease with extensive details of post-mortem examination, including histology. The prevalence of disease in specific parts of cities was documented. There was little about the newborn. Papers were often 20 pages in length that few modern readers would tolerate. Gradually the papers became shorter, and a short report section was added in 1970. In 1973 there were two annotations a year. In 1985 there were 24 annotations, with nine personal practice articles and ten current topic articles. This 'commissioned' section has expanded further and fills many of the ever increasing number of pages. By 2015 there were 2 editorials, 1–2 leading articles and 3–4 review articles in each edition. Reader surveys in 1993 showed that review articles were the most popular. These are still the most popular content evidenced by reader surveys, download statistics and direct feedback to the editorial team. There is so much potential content out there for readers to consider. This has increased exponentially with the advent of the World Wide Web. We are in 'competition' for the readers' time and so messages need to be clear, focussed, relevant and correct. Most readers read the contents column, a few summaries and a small number of articles in detail. Many readers will access the journal content through one of the common Internet search engines.

In the 1980s, there were rumours that the neonatologists were planning a new journal. We were not keen to have the competition of a new journal, because a large proportion of our readers practised both general paediatrics and neonatal medicine, and we would lose up to 50 % of our best papers. With the increasing clamour of the increasing number of neonatologists, the separate Fetal and Neonatal Edition was added in 1988. This has been a great success – now 6 editions per year, 96 pages and an impact factor greater than 3.0. The FNN edition mirrors the ADC edition with a combination of commissioned and submitted content. The journal has a team of specialist editors (although expertise is shared across all three editions) led by Martin Ward Platt and Ben Stenson as joint edition editors. All papers are still triaged by the editor-in-chief.

The main edition includes general and speciality content aiming for the wider paediatric readership with now specialist editors for most specialities. Papers from all areas are encouraged including epidemiology and public health, child psychiatry, adolescent medicine, community paediatrics and global child health. The journal has included a 3-month drug therapy section since 2009.

In the 1990s, a section in the contents list for community paediatrics was introduced to encourage research, but the number of submitted articles remained low. When the community paediatricians proposed a separate edition, that section was placed at the top of the contents page. Community paediatrics has evolved into the specialities of epidemiology, public health, neurodisability, education, child protection and social and behavioural disabilities. As the majority of paediatricians are interested in several of these subjects, the community section heading was deleted and the submitted and commissioned work listed with the other content.

The number of original articles submitted has increased year on year with more than 1000 submissions in 2015 and an acceptance rate of around 15 %.

It is a great challenge to decide how to select the best content. There have been perennial discussions on whether there should be one or two referees and whether they should be 'blind' to the identity of author. This is ongoing – everything still goes for 'blind peer review' and mostly two referees and statisticians if the article contains complex statistics and is then discussed at the editorial committee or 'hanging committee' as it was previously known. This is now mostly a teleconference rather than a face-to-face meeting – relevant and necessary with the increased complexity of articles submitted, increasing numbers of editors and internationalisation of the journal.

In the 1990s, the editorial board at its annual retreat repeatedly criticised the short reports as being anecdotal and of no scientific merit, although they provided important clinical reminders and were an opportunity for junior staff to start to write. This section was integrated with the standard research papers but later reappeared as short reports, case reports and images.

Empty space between articles was a constant criticism until it was filled by extracts from other journals wittily prepared by Doug Addy under the pseudonym 'Archivist'. Part of Archivist became Journal Watch and some of this white space is now used for images, notices and advertisements. Doug Addy wrote the page of short extracts at the end of the journal which he called 'Lucina' until 2012 when he retired. He was much missed and has been replaced by Robert Scott Jupp – who has continued the entertaining and occasionally controversial reporting of content from other journals.

There have been many innovations. The page for the editor-in-chief directs the reader to key papers in that edition as well as provides an opportunity for comment on the papers and is recorded as a monthly podcast. The perspectives section (now editorials) puts an original paper into the perspective of the literature but occasionally makes the reader wonder whether the paper should have been accepted for publication. The meticulous analysis of research would have delighted Barlow. An editorial is attractive to the reader, but it may be difficult to persuade a busy research worker to produce it timely and not hold up publication of the original article. There is an unethical temptation to accept a mediocre paper that will be savaged by the writer of the perspective; the ADC editor never succumbs!

The Archimedes section encourages a critical approach to practice based on the PICO approach whereby the author asks a relevant question and through a careful review of the literature appraises the evidence to get the best answer or at least a clinical bottom line based on their review of the quality of the published evidence.

When compulsory continuing professional development (CPD) was introduced 25 years ago, the editors met the academic board of the College and suggested that all review articles should be sent to a designated member of the Board who would recommend which, if any, should be approved for CPD. This agreement was never implemented. Education and Practice Edition was launched in 2014 with a mission 'to assist paediatricians at all levels in their training and ongoing professional development' [5]. There are now six editions a year, 60 pages each. All articles are commissioned – clinically focussed – an opportunity for young people to write and very popular with readers particularly with innovative content such as how to use, 15-min consultation, problem solving in clinical practice, research in paediatrics, pharmacy update and guideline review. All content is approved by the RCPCH for continuing professional development, and there are 'self-testing' questions at the end of every article.

There were repeated requests to change the name of the journal which sounded musty and archaic, but none of the suggested names were acceptable to the editorial board. When the American Medical Association changed the name of their paediatric journal to Archives of Pediatrics and Adolescent Medicine in 1994, the debate stopped. The discussion has resurfaced with the AMA journals now being rebranded including Archives of Paediatrics and Adolescent Medicine becoming JAMA Paediatrics.

In 1999, an authoritative speaker told the editorial board that within 5 years the paper edition would carry only review papers. Over the past 15 years, the proportion of review to original papers has increased although well over half of the submissions (and content) are original articles across a wide range of specialist areas.

Achievements

Barlow's dreams have become a reality. The journal has adopted new technology, become more friendly to the reader, embraced more objective approaches to assessment and criticism of papers and provided an alluring buffet of high quality papers. The Archives continues to have the highest impact factor compared to other paediatric journals in Europe and improved from 1.79 in 2005 to 2.65 in 2010 and 2.9 in 2014. The impact factor is the number of citations in other papers in one particular year divided by the number of articles published during the previous 2 years and is considered one of the best indicators of scientific quality. A paper published in a journal with a higher impact factor attracts a higher government research grant for the originating unit. More paediatricians are taking part in the editorial process that provides training. The number of submissions has increased from 1602 in 2005 to more than 2000 from 2010 with more than 50 % from outside the UK. The acceptance rate has been constant at about 15–20 % for original articles. The international board has encouraged papers and readers from a wider geographical area. Global child health papers are encouraged. There is now a monthly global child health section in the journal, and the journal hosted a millennium development goals meeting (and supplement) in early 2015 [8].

The explosion of information technology has expanded the journal reach, and there are now other markers of success than the impact factor including things like the 'PDF download rate' and Altmetric which looks at the impact of the article to the wider community – effectively as a marker of how much the article is likely to impact on practice – measured from such things as Twitter reach, Facebook impressions, blogs and number of news agencies that cover the content.

The Archives has been a major source of postgraduate education, but the development of 23 specialty groups in the College and the changing attitude to postgraduate education have made the editors' task more difficult. When Continuous Medical Education (CME) was introduced 15 years ago, the emphasis was on keeping up to date with all aspects of paediatrics and child health. After replacement by CPD, enhancing personal skills became the priority – a difficult goal for a general journal. Professor Howard Bauchner who was editor-in-chief of the Archives for 11 years until 2011 managed to achieve 'this difficult balance' [6] of getting the best content, maintaining the interest of the reader (generalist and specialist) and promoting education and training from his clinical base in Boston, USA. He has been appointed editor-in-chief of the Journal of the American Medical Association, one of the most prestigious medical journals in the world. This appointment is a recognition of the impressive achievements of Howard and his team at the Archives.

There are many challenges – the changing world of publication, the explosion of journals, the complexities of open access, the need to disseminate research, the complexities of implementation science, the importance of quality improvement, the explosion in the social media and promoting the content post publication, but the mission of the journal remains as at its inception – to inform and educate paediatricians about new and relevant research that can impact their practice and thereby improve the care of children.

Professor RM Beattie is the current editor-in-chief of Archives of Disease in Childhood.

References

1. Lock SP. For wrapping fish and chips? Arch Dis Child. 1986;61:966–8.
2. Anonymous. The archives of disease in childhood. BMJ. 1926;1:209–10.
3. Moncrieff A. The British Paediatric Association. In: Cameron HC, editor. 1928–1952. p. 102–7.
4. Barlow T. Introduction. Arch Dis Child. 1926;1:1–6.
5. Blair M. Getting evidence into practice: implementation science for paediatricians. Arch Dis Child. 2014;99(4):307–9.
6. Bauchner H, McIntosh N, Editorial. Arch Dis Child Educ Pract Ed. 2004;89:1–2.
7. Lock SP. A difficult balance. London: The Nuffield Provincial Hospitals Trust; 1985.
8. Millennium development goals progress report. Arch Disease Child. 2015;S1:1–80.

The Annual Meeting

22

Rosalind Topping, Graham Clayden, Alan Craft,
Dennis Gill, Alun Elias-Jones, David Walker,
and Ricky Richardson

An annual gathering of members has been held since the early days of the BPA. Indeed the size of the membership was for many years determined by the capacity of the dining room at the Old England Hotel in Windermere. For many members this annual getting together was their sole contact with their association/ college. The founders of the BPA were adamant that one of the main purposes of getting professionals together was that of camaraderie. The social events which have largely occurred at the annual meetings have been most important occasions with which to pursue this aim. In Chap. 4 Andrew Wilkinson has described the first annual meeting after the formation of the College. Rosalind Topping who organised these meetings for over 25 years here reflects on them.

The scientific programme has in recent years consisted of plenary and parallel group sessions of the specialty groups. With the growth of the number of such groups and the shortage of space, there has often been a need for 'doubling up'. There are several named guest lectures which have been given by some of the world's most

R. Topping • G. Clayden • R. Richardson
London, UK

A. Craft (✉)
Newcastle, UK

D. Gill
Dublin, Ireland

A. Elias-Jones
Leicester, UK

D. Walker
Nottingham, UK

© Springer International Publishing Switzerland 2017
A. Craft, K. Dodd (eds.), *From an Association to a Royal College*,
DOI 10.1007/978-3-319-43582-4_22

distinguished paediatricians and others with an interest in children. The latest two chief medical officers, Sir Liam Donaldson and Dame Sally Davies, have addressed the meeting.

Planning for the meeting starts at least 2 years before the event and booking of the venue at least 5 years. For many years, the venue was the University campus at York, but in recent years it has rotated around the UK.

Members and their guests are encouraged to submit abstracts of their work, and the best are chosen for plenary presentation and the remainder offered to the specialty groups for their sessions. In recent years, there have been stunning presentations from medical students as well as established paediatricians. Many of today's academic leaders gave their first major conference presentations at the annual meeting.

The quality of the presentations has improved dramatically over the years. 25 years ago presentations were illustrated by slides; it was not uncommon for them to be illegible, and the standard of presentation could sometimes be challenging. Today we have PowerPoint, and most presentations are of a really high standard with legible illustrations and presenters stick to time.

The Annual Meeting Reflections of Rosalind Topping

'*April 1997 sees the first Annual Scientific Meeting of the Royal College of Paediatrics and Child Health, which owes everything to its forbear, the BPA. The College has inherited a robust foundation of democratic representation, vigour, commitment, loyalty, tradition, friendship and fun*'. These sentiments, expressed by Professor Sir Roy Meadow, President, still hold true today.

Since then, membership numbers have trebled; the number of papers presented at the meeting has grown, as has the number and variety of sessions; and attendance numbers have gone up. Alongside these general movements, a number of highlights stand out.

In 1997, the College cut its teeth on the organisation of royal visits. HRH, the Princess Royal, our Patron, attended a plenary session in which she presented the James Spence medal and certificates to the newly elected Honorary Fellows, addressed the audience and engaged with members informally over coffee. This set a pattern for return visits in the following years.

Another memorable feature that year was a multi-faith service of thanksgiving in York Minster. The sharp-eyed would have noted trainees, seated side by side on a pew, serendipitously representing the world's major ethnic groups and religions.

The Annual Dinner moved to York racecourse in 1997. It was followed by a spectacular firework display from the grandstand which resulted in a visit from the police the next morning. In the absence of advance warning about this noisy spectacle, the good citizens of York had telephoned them in a state of consternation and alarm.

A memory from 1998 to 1999 is of President Professor David Baum handing an apple to each plenary-free paper presenter, with a special memento when it coincided with 1 April. A tradition of joyous dancing after the Annual Dinner took off in 1998 to music provided by the Back Seat Jivers, a jazz band led by Steve Salfield, a College Fellow.

In 1999 there were dramatic changes, with the first customised stage set and the registration area professionally dressed, so as to lift the impact of the space and boldly stamp it with the College's identity.

The millennium was marked by a series of special lectures and a firework display on the campus, which this time passed off without incident. The University of York set their audio-visual standards by those required by the College. The 2003 George Frederic Still Memorial Lecture challenged the technicians' skill, however, with the biggest data file they had up to that point ever loaded onto their system, and this was handed to them one hour before the start of the lecture.

The SPARKS Young Investigator of the Year, Paul Polani and Tony Jackson awards were all initiated in the last 15 years, and 2011 saw the first David Harvey Fellowship given for a health professional working to improve child health in a disadvantaged part of the world.

In 2010, the conference moved back to the University of Warwick, the first in a series of changes intended to shape the conference to meet the present needs of the diversity of paediatricians who attend, and to provide them with inspirational ideas to take home.

The Scottish Paediatric Society's 90th anniversary was celebrated at the 2012 Annual Conference in Glasgow.

There has always been a well-visited trade exhibition growing in size and in recent years has had charity and other exhibitors.

One of the highlights of the annual meeting has been the concerts played by a scratch orchestra largely comprised of paediatricians who have brought their instruments along to the meeting and had intensive rehearsals resulting in quite outstanding concerts. Graham Clayden, paediatrician at St Thomas's, has largely been responsible for this activity.

Music at York, Graham Clayden

There were two factors that spawned the idea of a scratch orchestra and choir to perform at the Annual Meetings. Graham Clayden and Joe Meyer had discovered that their midlife crisis response had been to take up the bassoon and then they had played together in secret at the Annual Meeting in the late 1980s. The second was the popularity of the regular annual professional musical evening performance. Why not meet this need for passive audience musical reception with the opportunity for paediatricians to share their musical skills however rudimentary? At the time there were a number of schisms within the BPA such as the division of opinion about the wisdom of splitting from the RCPs and, more emotionally, the difficulties around paediatricians' management of suspected child abuse. What better way than music to shelve differences – not quite rerunning the Christmas trenches' ceasefire for carols and football but an attempt to all sing from the same song sheet.

The first event was in 1990 when a gathering of keen but very mixed-ability paediatricians offered excerpts from Handel's Messiah conducted intermittently by Andrew Porter swinging his clarinet to establish an agreed beat. As recorded in the newsletter/flyer to recruit musicians for the 1991 meeting, 'the inaugural performance....was perceived then as a social if not a complete musical success'. Undeterred, even when the BPA Annual Meeting Planning Committee refused to replace the professional chamber concert with this newborn paediatric endeavour, plans were made to gather as much of the musical talent within the BPA as we could muster and put on a much more professional attempt. After all, most paediatricians have been pleasantly surprised by the amazing progress of newborns who had appeared very weak at birth. It was this 1991 concert that won the confidence of the BPA hierarchy and the support of the membership. John Maclaurin not only astounded everyone with his mastery of Mozart Piano Concerto K488 but found us Budoc Goudie as our first professional conductor.

The 1992 concert allowed the choral singers their chance to startle their colleagues as well as to celebrate the composer's 236th birthday by performing most parts of Mozart Requiem. By 1993 the shape of the informal gathering that was to last 16 years became established. Keeping our paediatric nature paramount, we were led by James Ross the son of a prominent paediatrician and accompanied through the few rehearsals and performances on the organ by the paediatrician and gifted composer John Ellis. Our constraints were the number of rehearsals possible from members from all around the UK and beyond, making it impossible to arrange rehearsals prior to the meeting. Also the main reason for paediatricians to come was the scientific meeting with its very packed agenda, leaving few opportunities for attendance by all eventual performers at any one rehearsal. By convincing the BPA of our audience-pleasing capacity, we were able to access some of the funds that would have paid for the professional chamber group to pay for some filler parts of the orchestra when vitally needed or to aid moral/musical support to our players. James Ross proved a genius at both matching the programme with our musical level and limited rehearsal potential and drawing out the innate talent with such humour and sympathy. The table lists the programmes over the years that cover the range that was possible with our limited rehearsal time, and it was also a great opportunity to try out the new compositions by John Ellis and be joined by performances of other than western music. When the BPA blossomed into the RCPCH, our President David Baum, who had been a strong supporter during our formation, commissioned a choral and instrumental work – An Heritage of the Lord based on Psalm 127, the motto to the college, by the composer Nicholas Ansdell-Evans which was performed with great acclaim.

BPA/RCPCH Annual Meeting Concerts

1990: Handel, *Messiah* (sections)

1991: Mozart, *Piano concerto K488*

1992: Mozart, *Requiem*

1993: Schubert, *5th Symphony*

1994: Mozart, *Ave Verum Corpus*; Schubert, Symphony No. 3; Mozart, *Requiem*.

1995: Beethoven, Symphony No. 1; Handel, *Messiah* (sections).

1996: Gibbons, *The Silver Swan*; Mozart, Symphony No. 25; Haydn, *The Creation* (sections).

1997: Haydn, Symphony No. 90; Bruckner, *Locus iste*; Fauré, *Requiem*.

1998: Haydn, Symphony No. 90; John Ellis, *Psalm 118* (first performance); Nicholas Ansdell-Evans, Cantata: *An Heritage of the Lord* (first performance).

1999: J. Strauss, Thunder and Lightning Polka; Fauré, Cantique de Jean Racine; Vivaldi, Gloria; Ansdell-Evans, An Heritage of the Lord.

2000: Vivaldi, Concerto in G minor RV 103; Haydn, *Nelson Mass*.

2001: Handel, Judas Maccabaeus

2002: Ravel, Pavane pour une infante défunte; John Ellis, Care-Charmer Sleep (first performance); Haydn, Te Deum (Marie Thérèse)

2003: Shostakovich, 2nd Waltz, Jazz Suite No. 2; Bruckner: *Afferentur regi*; *Locus iste*; *Vexilla regis*; Mozart, *Coronation Mass*. Professor Sverre Lie an Honorary Fellow from Oslo played Greig's 'Wedding breakfast at Trolldhagen'

2004: John Ellis, *Two Poems by Mattie Stepacek* (first performance); excerpts from Handel, *Solomon*

2005: Haydn, *The Season* (excerpts)

2006: Fauré, *Pavane*; Tippett, Spirituals: *A Child of Our Time*; Mozart, *Requiem* (excerpts)

2007: Mozart, Posthorn Serenade; JS Bach, Magnificat in D

2009: Byrd, Ave Verum Corpus; JS Bach, Air: Orchestral Suite No. 3; Mozart, Ave Verum Corpus; Mozart, Divertimento in F, K. 213; Bruckner, Locus iste; Elgar, Ave Verum Corpus.

Over the years the orchestra and choir have had members from all branches of paediatrics and a wide range of experience. A number of the medical students who attended as nominees from their universities have joined in, as have a growing number of honorary and retired fellows.

Since 2000 the numbers in the choir and orchestra have dropped as a result of increasing time pressure that prevents many members and fellows attending the full Annual Meeting. The sad death of John Ellis had a major impact on our ability to rehearse and has robbed us of our depth of musical talent. However this musical group fulfils one of the statutes of the RCPCH Royal Charter, that is, to promote fellowship amongst paediatricians, and so we have great confidence in the survival of our group in one form or another.

The BPA Marathon Trophy

Alan Craft

In 1982 the first London Marathon took place shortly before the Annual Meeting in York. At least two members, George Rylance and Alan Craft, turned up in York proudly wearing their hard-earned medals. As an inspiration to other would-be marathon runners, they persuaded Wyeth to sponsor a BPA marathon trophy to be awarded at the Annual Dinner to the paediatrician who had run the fastest marathon anywhere during that year. Over the next few years, the names of Craft and Rylance were the most prominent in winning the magnificent trophy until time crept up on them, and they gave way to the much younger, and faster, Angus Nichol.

Sadly, although marathon running remains very popular, even amongst paediatricians, the trophy is no longer awarded.

Golf: The Ulster Cup, Dennis Gill

The Ulster Cup, so named because it was donated to the BPA in 1935 when the Association met in Newcastle, County Down, is a hotly contested golf trophy open to BPA/now RCPCH members. For many paediatricians, winning the Ulster Cup (a beautiful silver trophy) is akin to a 'major' and draws applause and acclaim when presented at the Annual Dinner. The first competition was played at the Royal County Down Golf Club, still amongst the finest links courses in the world. Since then, the Ulster Cup (80 years old in 2015) has been played close to the annual meeting venue, in Windermere, York, (Fulford and Ganton GCs), Warwick, Birmingham, etc., by, unfortunately, dwindling numbers in recent years.

The most frequent winner has been Jim Littlewood of Leeds (3½ times), Robyn Cain (3 times), Clive Ryder (3 times), two different Nick Barnes' (twice each) and Peter Dunn (1½ times) – he and Jim Littlewood must have eschewed the customary countback for draws. Other notable winning names include Alex Campbell and Bertie Webb. I believe that an NI paediatrician has yet to win the Ulster Cup, though four ROI 'paediatricians' (Brian McNicholl, Seamus O'Donoghue, Denis Gill, Alf Nicholson) have been successful. Former president Terence Stephenson has competed on a number of occasions.

Clive Ryder has organised the competition in the twenty-first century, preceded by Dr. Reynolds. The Ulster Cup competition was not held in 2014. Hopefully the Ulster Cup will survive as a golf competition, a source of companionship and a worthy RCPCH venture.

Squash

The Schlesinger-Dent Squash Tournament.
Alun Elias-Jones

From 1960, at the Annual Meeting of the BPA and then RCPCH, a knockout squash rackets tournament was held for consultant members and fellows, and the winner received the Schlesinger-Dent trophy which had originated from University College Hospital. In 1987, a senior registrar Alun Elias-Jones who happened to be a Welsh international player was allowed to participate. Thereafter anyone attending the conference including overseas visitors and guests were invited to play. The players varied in standard from club players to county players and other former internationals, such as Dr. Neil Martin, a former Scottish international. Several players won it more than one time including Roy Harris, Jeff Bissenden and Huw Jenkins. Alun Elias-Jones, a Welsh international, won it 15 times. The rule was that the winner had to organise the event the following year which led to a degree of continuity. The tournament was last held in 2006.

In recent years since approximately 2000 with competing activities and members, concerns about continual professional development as the number of players entering declined the format changed to a round robin league with the two players winning the most matches contesting the final the following day. Although played in a friendly spirit, a lady player did on one occasion break her leg and had to be driven back to London by the college lawyer Bertie Leigh. Fortunately no claim for compensation was made! The players would follow the squash with a social trip to one of the campus bars to rehydrate and have a buffet supper.

Speed Croquet
David Walker and Ricky Richardson

2010 and 2011 saw the RCPCH venture into the sport of kings: speed croquet. In 2010 a small band of devotees tested their skills on the lawns of Warwick. The idea was to have a pleasant game, share good company and raise a little money. Ricky Richardson had mentored the Sultan of Brunei on the croquet lawn. David Walker had developed a speed version to mix his researchers up.

All was developing nicely in Warwick in 2010; a select few participated one lunchtime. The winners recorded in the winter newsletter were Russell Viner paired with Alistair Scammell. In 2011 all was set for an end-of-day game; we enjoyed a bigger turnout, drinks were served, but no record was made of the winner that day, although a prize was awarded at dinner by President Terence Stephenson. We set our sights on Glasgow for 2012 but found the nearest croquet lawn too far from our venue to be practical.

So what next? The game is perfect for paediatricians in need of social recreation with an edge. The speed version allows 16 people to play at once for 10 min or so offering a setting for up to 80 people to play in an hour on a single lawn, although the organisation would need to be dynamic and the alcohol limited to get that level of cooperation. Will it rise again? Should we select the conference venue by the availability of a suitable lawn? We leave the challenge to others to make this work in years to come.

Olympic Success

Two gold medals were won at the Rio Olympics in 2016 by offspring of College members. Alastair Brownlee, son of Keith in the triathlon and Owain Doull, son of Iolo, in the cycling.

The Annual General Meeting – Social events (The orchestra)

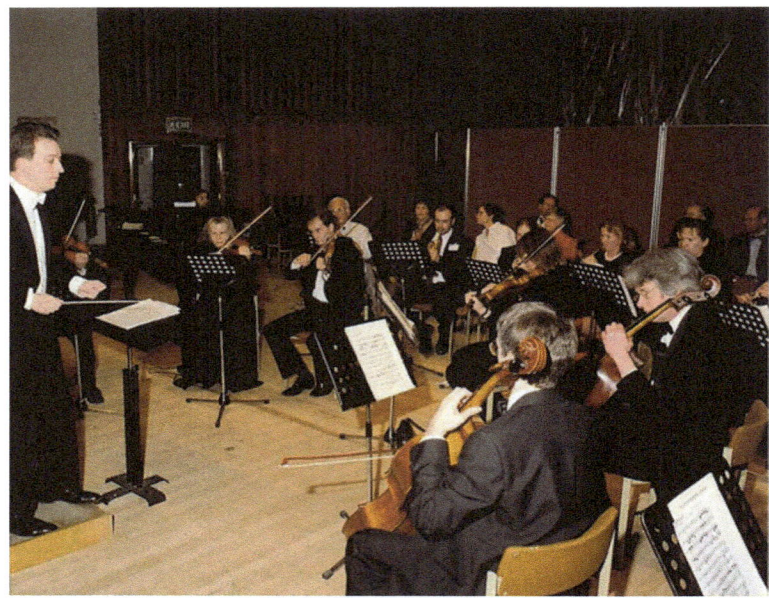

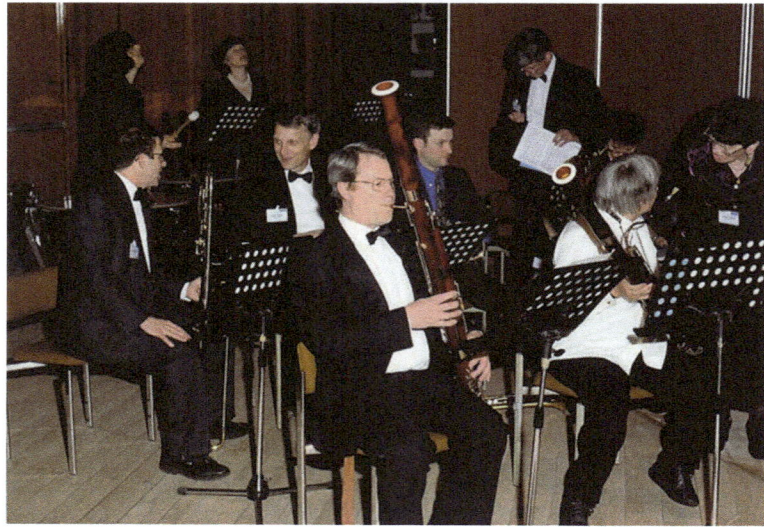

The Annual General Meeting – Social events (The choir and orchestra)

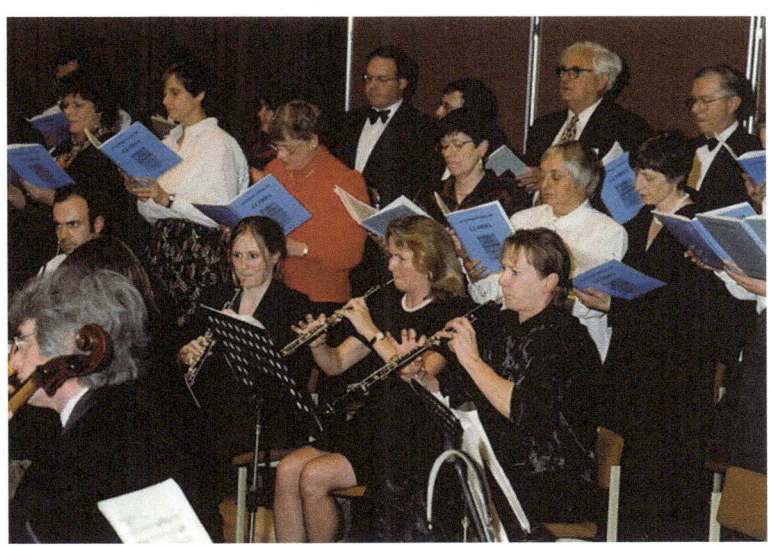

Medical students relaxing

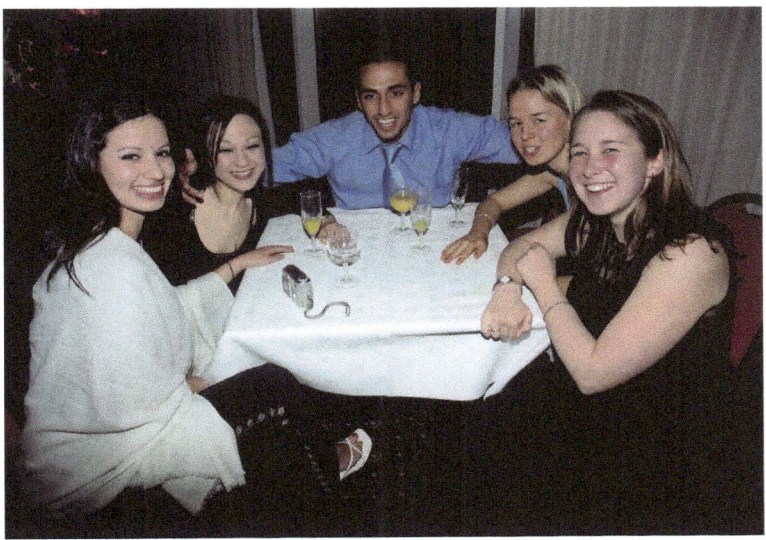

Steve Salfield with the "Back Seat Jivers"

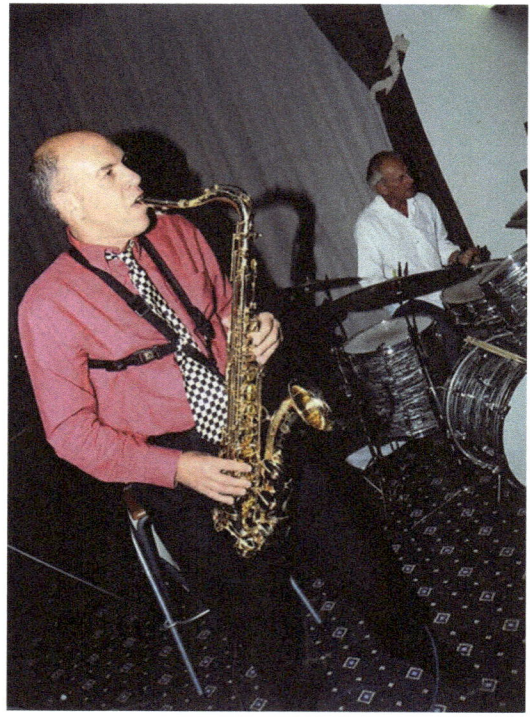

Janet Anderson

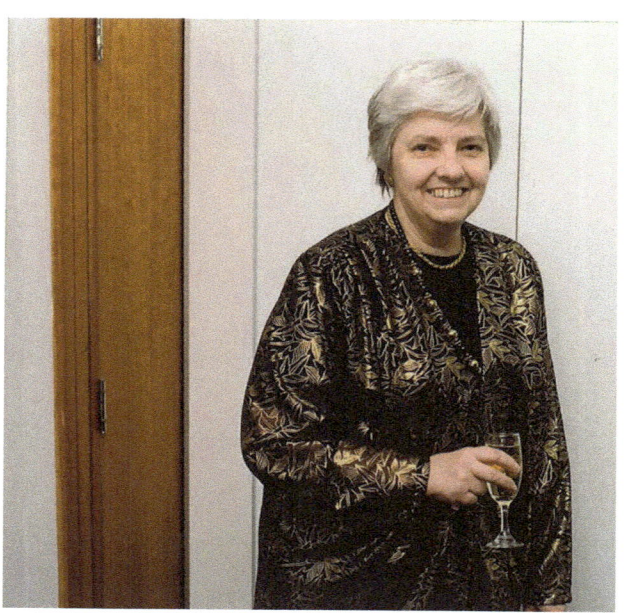

Rosalind Topping and Amanda Ambalu, conference organisers

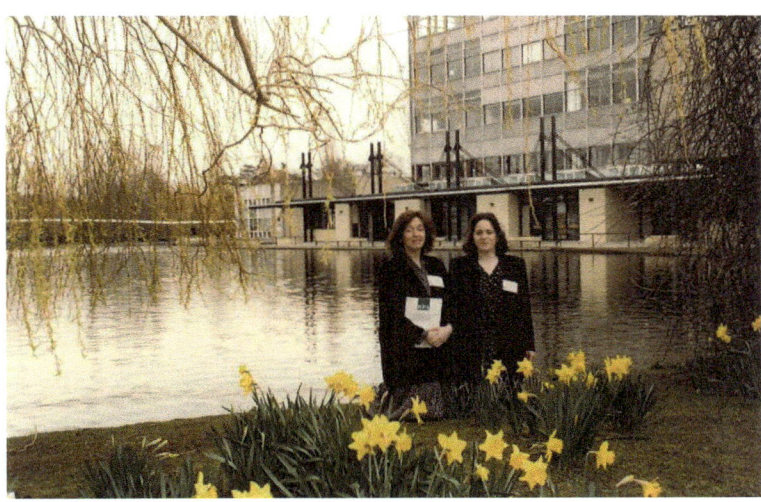

David Baum and June Lloyd

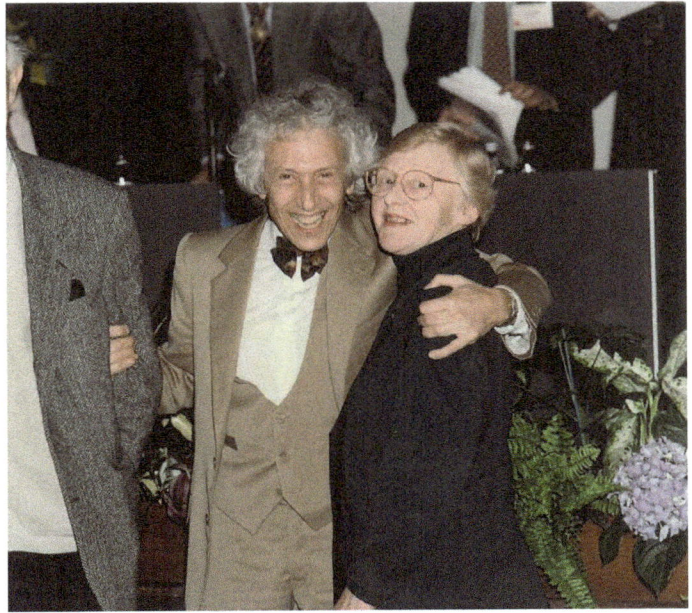

Professors John Forfar and Otto Wolff

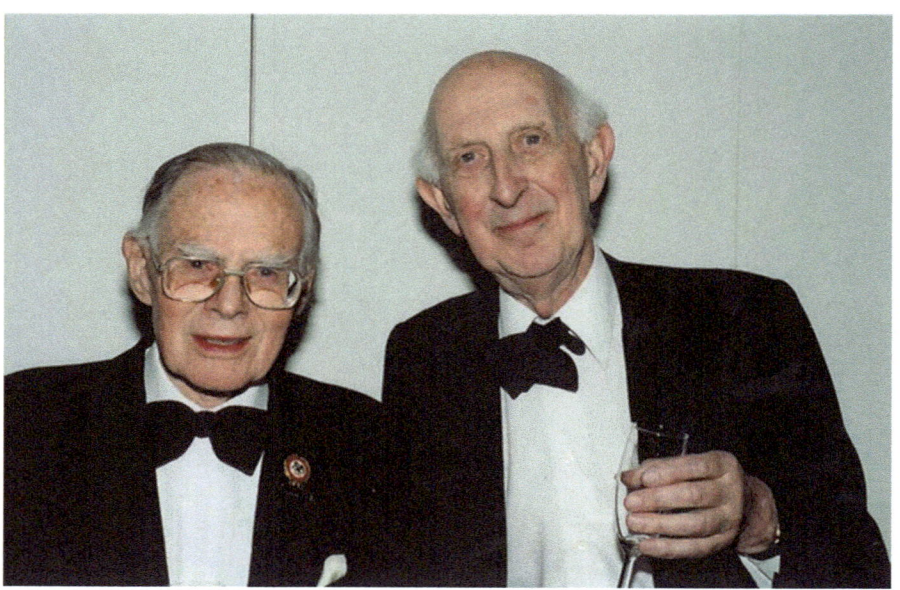

College Secretaries and Chief Executive Officers

23

Paul Dunn, James Kempton, Len Tyler, Chris Hanvey, and Judith Ellis

The span of this history covers the terms of five college secretaries/chief executive officers, each of whom served under more than one president and played a critical part in the birth and early development of the college.

Paul Dunn steered the BPA over many years towards the transition to a college, and James Kempton guided us through the period of its foundation. Len Tyler settled the college in its new home and oversaw a period of rapid expansion as we took on the several new responsibilities of a college. More recently Chris Hanvey has revised the college staffing structure and broadened the college's outlook, and Judith Ellis is now leading on the modernisation of the college's governance structure and extending the college's reach, influence and impact on child health.

Paul Dunn

I was privileged to be Secretary of the BPA from January 1988 to July 1995.

These were years of rapid change; membership of the BPA was expanding, and staff numbers had to rise to cope. The office was housed throughout in premises rented from the RCPL at 5 St Andrew's Place, charming to look at, but designed for residential rather than office use. Our landlord kindly agreed to build more rooms in the well at the back, but this relief was only temporary. When I retired, the search for larger, modern premises was already on, and the move to 50 Hallam Street followed.

P. Dunn • J. Kempton • L. Tyler • J. Ellis (✉) • C. Hanvey
London, UK

© Springer International Publishing Switzerland 2017
A. Craft, K. Dodd (eds.), *From an Association to a Royal College*,
DOI 10.1007/978-3-319-43582-4_23

In 1988 (Jubilee year for the BPA), we had no Internet. Word processors were coming in, but communication between officers, members and the office was by phone and post. Nobody had a website. Agenda and minutes travelled by mail, or courier within inner London. Most members paid subscriptions by cheque, a few by standing order. Direct debit was regarded by many with deep suspicion. I remember negotiating with the bank manager to transfer any surplus BPA cash automatically to a deposit account each evening. The Auditor to the BPA was literally a one-man band. The modest surplus accumulated from 1928 to 1988 was invested cautiously, gaining 2.5 % interest, and the Hon Treasurer was not yet supported by a Finance Committee.

As staff numbers began to rise, the question of a contributory staff pension scheme had to be tackled; a short-list of possible companies was drawn up, and presentations were made to the Finance Committee.

The presidents I served under were Professors Forfar, Lloyd, Hull and Meadow. It was an education to me to observe how hard they all worked, as did all the officers. This was particularly so during the Butler Sloss enquiry, the MMR vaccine controversy and the Clothier enquiry.

Meetings took place at the DoH between BPA officers and politicians such as William Waldegrave and Virginia Bottomley. It is my personal belief that the high quality of these discussions helped the BPA cause a few years later when the application for a college became official.

The Jubilee service in Westminster Abbey was arranged through a member, General Sir Alan Reay; the special BPA exhibition in the House of Commons was made possible by Barry Sherman MP. Both helped to raise the BPA profile. So too did the series of presidential dinners. Another useful aid were special publications, such as 'Child Health in a Changing Society' (OUP 1988) and the third volume of the history of the BPA. The printer of the latter amazed us by his wizardry with computer technology, taking a variety of faded sepia photographs from the BPA's photo albums and somehow producing crisp b/w headshots in a consistent format. Later came the facsimile reproduction of 'The Boke of Chyldren' by Thomas Phaire.

At the end of the 1980s, the venue for the BPA's spring meeting changed from York to Warwick; this called for extra effort by Rosalind Topping and team, who rose to the challenge with typical aplomb.

The various referenda held on the issue of a college were administered by the Electoral Reform Society; it was an education for me to meet the ERS and to learn how they operate. Further education arose when I accompanied the officers and Mr Leigh of Hempsons to the preliminary meeting with the clerk to the Privy Council. There followed much drafting of documents with Hempsons and much lobbying.

My contract of employment specified retirement at age 60; hence, I stepped down some 6 months before the Privy Council gave the go-ahead. The college kindly appointed Mr Leigh and I as honorary fellows.

James Kempton

I was lucky enough and immensely proud to be associated with the BPA/RCPCH at probably the most significant moment in its history: as the last Secretary of the BPA, the only ever Secretary of the College of Paediatrics and Child Health, and first Secretary of the RCPCH. That period gave me great personal satisfaction and experiences that come only once – if indeed ever – in any career. I have some unforgettable memories!

Most Memorable Trip

My diary just says *9.30 am 11 December 1997, Buckingham Palace.* My memory is of a wide-eyed minicab driver trying to drop us off near the Victoria Memorial and not quite believing it when the gates of Buckingham Palace swung open to admit his rather clapped out saloon. He was not the only one feeling a little awestruck that day as David Baum, Keith Dodd and I were ushered into a private audience with Princess Anne in her sitting room somewhere upstairs in the Palace. David as ever was the one to break the ice: Beckoned by the Princess to sit beside her, he arrived there by flying across the room in true Marx Brothers style having tripped over the head of a huge polar bearskin rug. Fortunately no lasting damage was done to the rug, nor to the Princess nor her relationship with the college! Fortunately the first ever royal visit to the college's offices in Hallam St, where I found myself responsible for everything from security to buying suitable china for tea, was a great success.

First Impressions

Coming from another medical royal college, I remember the culture shock of joining an organisation that seemed at the time less like an institution and more like a members club. The culture was decidedly paternalistic. The small staff team comprised many highly experienced and long-serving people like Rosalind Topping as well as newer arrivals like Aaron Barham. The main duty of the secretary (head of paid staff) seemed to be opening every piece of correspondence that came into the building and deciding what should happen to it. Rather than acting as strategic leader, as I had been used to. The honorary officers functioned more like departmental managers making day-to-day decisions and directly managing staff. It was a model of working that people were attached to and one that had served the BPA well. While there was acceptance that this culture could not survive the increased complexity and staff team that would come with the anticipated (but not yet confirmed) college status, developing a vision and consensus about how the college would operate in the future featured throughout my period as secretary.

Not all my memories are good ones and even now I am still haunted by the nightmare that was IT. It did not start well, with a brand new system that no one seemed to have confidence in and which was struggling to perform the absolutely essential task of collecting the monthly subscriptions much to the frustration of the membership administrator, Andy Becker. But then things got decidedly worse when a disgruntled member of staff made an attempt at sabotage. Inevitably many of the memories would only mean something to the people who were there at the time like all the staff sitting in the basement tired and dirty and eating pizza with Tracey Guest and Philippa Davies having finally finished packing up and moving out of St Andrew's Place; Sir Roy Meadow handing out £100 cheques to staff to celebrate finally getting college status; trying to work out what on earth you did with a Royal Charter when it turned up and subsequently choosing the right frame to last for posterity; waving RCPCH placards to direct groups of people into the magnificent service in York Minster at 6.15 on 17 April 1997 which celebrated the First Annual Meeting of the RCPCH. What It Means to Be a College. A lot of what I remember most clearly was in effect all about what sort of institution the college would be and what symbols would be used to describe that to the rest of the world. Much of that debate as I look back on it seems to have been between the traditionalists and modernisers: portraits (yes), mace (yes), coat of arms or logo (coat of arms), patron (yes), royal or someone worthy by achievement rather than birth (royal). My childhood enthusiasm for heraldry was now so relevant a skill that I wondered why I had omitted to put it on my job application. So I guess you would conclude that it was a debate the traditionalists won.

Over and above issues around pageantry was the question of our new HQ: how much space did we need and how much could we afford to spend? Getting away from the overshadowing presence of the RCP was a given, but the debate about functional and modern over learned and institutional was something which as secretary I took a keen interest in. When I arrived in 1996, the secretary managed 17 administrators and 6 staff in the research unit led by Jon Pollock. But John Osborne, the Hon Treasurer, was nervously looking at the affordability of staffing estimates of as many as 50 staff over the coming 5 years. As it turned out the college grew rather modestly over my time as secretary with the massive increase coming later.

So while staff numbers and responsibilities grew with becoming a college, for me the greatest challenge, and for the staff the greatest change, came from moving to a new building. Walking into the Medical Protection Society's former HQ at 50 Hallam St, I think we all immediately got that 'this is the one for us' feeling. The location was well known to anyone interested in medicine because it was next door to the then home of the GMC. Compared to our accommodation in St Andrew's Place and the new temporary satellite offices across Regent's Park in Cornwall Terrace, it offered a council chamber, great offices for staff and space for members and meetings. It was imposing without being grandiose and had more than enough space for the college to grow into over time. The MPS settled for a fair price and were extremely generous in the fixtures, fittings and office furniture they left behind, so we looked the part in our new home too. Definitely a job well done!

Conclusion

My leaving present was a pair of gold RCPCH-crested cuff links which I wear with great pride. I have gone on to serve children and young people in other ways, as a teacher and as a politician and policy maker, but I have continued to watch the college's progress with interest and affection.

Len Tyler

I joined RCPCH as secretary in June 1998. The college had just obtained its royal charter and moved into new premises in Hallam Street. Though we were a medical royal college in name, however, many of the key functions still had to be put into place – in particular we had to take over the running of our examinations from the RCP. We also lacked much of the infrastructure we now take for granted. There was no IT department; HR was handled on a part-time basis by the secretary's office – as was press work (aided very capably by Dr Harvey Marcovitch) and publications. There was certainly no archivist – files from the old offices had been brought over and piled into the basement of Hallam Street, waiting for somebody to sort them into some kind of order. We still had only about 30 staff and the secretary's job was very much hands on. I remember during my first few weeks helping carry tables and chairs to prepare for a council meeting and even sitting on the switchboard for a couple of hours when the receptionist went sick and nobody else was available.

The first step was a restructuring of college departments. A new exams department was created almost immediately. We also set up a small IT section. HR and press calls remained for the moment with the secretary, however, and the files in the basement lay undisturbed for some time.

The next 10 years were ones of heady and almost continuous growth. Examinations work expanded rapidly, and exams fees soon provided about a third of our income. Our research work grew too, funded mainly by external grants. Continuous professional development also attained a much higher profile. Our press and parliamentary work also became a lot more important, and we appointed our first full-time press officer. This last was part of our growing public profile. The media came to us more and more for comments. Meetings with government ministers, which had previously been quite rare, now became routine. We also routinely met opposition spokesmen and were able to have a number of meetings with Andrew Lansley to gauge what the health policy of the next government would be. International work was something else that needed to be started almost from scratch. Three international director posts were set up to oversee work in different parts of the world, and an international committee was established. We tried from the start to give long-term help to a few areas rather than spread ourselves too thinly. The projects in the West Bank and Gaza, led by Dr Tony Waterston, achieved considerable success.

Staff numbers expanded accordingly. The Hallam Street building, which had initially seemed far larger than we could possibly need – we had contemplated turning over the entire ground floor as a cafeteria – quickly filled up. We rented additional floors in the building next door and then the whole space, knocking through on the ground floor and basement levels. We also took on a floor of a building in Great Portland Street for the research division. The long search for a more permanent solution to our space problems began. One near miss was a converted church in Pentonville Road. We also spent a lot of time negotiating with the GMC on the possible purchase of their lease once they had moved to Euston Road. Eventually we settled on Theobalds Road, at that time undergoing a refit. We sold Hallam Street, giving ourselves the deadline of Easter 2008 for moving out of one building and into the other. Easter Sunday saw the (now) Chief Executive of RCPCH back in hands-on mode, helping to carry boxes as we completed the move on time and, remarkably, within budget. The process had been surprisingly smooth, one of the most heated debates being, when it came to designing new letterheads, over whether there was an apostrophe in 'Theobalds'. (We decided there wasn't.)

The expansion of our functions called for a second major restructuring of staff and committees. Staff numbers had grown to over 100, including those in the newly opened offices in Edinburgh and Cardiff. A new staffing structure was put in just before the move to Theobalds Road, setting up three new director posts coordinating, respectively, operations, internal services and policy. The positioning of research within this new structure – and how closely it should be linked to policy – remained a matter for debate that was not resolved until after my time. The restructuring of committees was trickier. It was relatively easy to agree a new strategic role for council and to reduce the size of EC and make it into a more responsive body for day-to-day decisions that could not be delegated elsewhere. Reducing the overall number of committees, something everyone agreed in principle was necessary, took much longer, and again was still in process when I left.

I worked for a number of presidents over the 11 years – David Baum, Richard Cooke (as acting president after David's sad death), David Hall, Alan Craft, Patricia Hamilton and Terence Stephenson. The relationship between the CEO and the president was always a key one for the college, and I was fortunate to coincide with a series of presidents who were far sighted and easy to work with. I am grateful to them and to the other officers and to the team of staff who worked for me.

Chris Hanvey

Coming to the RCPCH in February 2010 felt like stepping on the shoulders of giants. The college was well ensconced in Theobalds Road, with a staff group of about 115 and combined income of just over £9 M.

Organic growth amongst the staff team meant that some reorganisation was necessary, through the formation of four new divisions similar to that of other colleges. RCPCH now has a research and policy, education and training, corporate services and communications divisions. At the same time, the position of international work was strengthened by Professor Steve Allen's appointment as David Baum Fellow and Chair of the strengthened international committee.

To accompany the new staff structure, council also approved new mission and values statements and some rebranding, which both recognised the college's past and also provided a refocused image.

The college's influence continued to grow, under the president, Professor Terence Stephenson, who helped place the college at the centre of debates about reconfiguration and the proposed far-reaching changes to the health services. Being the default position for radio, TV and print media, comments on child health was assisted by a new media team and a new public affairs post, charged with ensuring that the college was a genuinely 'Four Nations' college. In 2011, the college was present, for the first time, at all three of the party conferences, lobbying Ministers and MPs to ensure that the health of children remained firmly on the agenda.

Spring 2011 saw the launch of a new website design, which aimed to make the college's Internet presence more accessible to all members. In autumn 2011, this was further enhanced by the college's Twitter feed.

The college also started to hold regular policy breakfasts to which government ministers were pleased to come, further putting the college at the centre of child health, at the heart of formulating policy in all four nations.

Judith Ellis

I was delighted to be appointed as Chief Executive of the college in September 2014 at which time the college membership had reached 16,000 and the budget was around £20 million.

It was an interesting induction as within 3 days of commencing in post, an EGM had rejected a proposal from the then president, Hilary Cass, to restructure the college to create a smaller Board of Trustees that included lay members to preserve a paediatrician representative council and create a multi-professional foundation. The emotion of the situation was in fact a unique opportunity for me as the new CEO. A restructuring of the Board of Trustees was required to meet Charity Commission's best practice, and, having not been involved prior to the EGM, to move the governance restructure forward, I needed to understand concerns and wishes. I therefore embarked on a 'UK tour' to actually ask members what they saw as an acceptable governance structure for their college and indeed what they wanted including in a 5-year college strategy. Attendance at this first round of open meetings varied widely, but themes were consistent. All accepted the vital role of the college in the education of trainees and for some CPD, but members had a limited knowledge of wider college activity in relation to child health. This insight and information led to the shared development of a new vision, strategy and operational plan that heightens activity to educate and involve the wider membership, including capitalising on the advocacy role of paediatricians through media and political activity. The college has over time been producing a suite of standards, guidance, guidelines and educational opportunities to support members in improving the care of infants, children and young people and, in times of austerity and vast changes in the NHS, the review and development of child health services. The focus now is to get these resources widely used for maximum impact! This includes not only the use by paediatricians but also all professionals and indeed increasingly empowering the children, young people and families themselves. The College are maximising on the power and spread of modern technology. Examples include: MindEd and Disability Matters, online educational packages which have been developed for professionals and lay access; best practice learning sites; and indeed Paediatric Care Online UK, a clinical decision-making tool with ever increasing access to high-quality supportive information for all professionals caring for children.

At the centre of our new vision are the infants, children, young people and families, and advocacy for child health is now at the core of all our activity. The College has developed the &Us network to innovatively use social media to actively engage with children, young people and parents and carers from across the UK. The RCPCH engagement leads collaborative has also been created to provide a virtual network for consultation and powerful child health political advocacy. The college now includes children and young people as committee members and indeed in 2016 for the first time invited young people to run the college for a day in a Takeover Challenge. It's worrying how well they did!

The impact of the College is ever increasing across the UK and also internationally. A new international board oversees the spread of college involvement. This includes worldwide education of paediatricians, partnership exchange, education activity to improve child health outcomes and through money from the David Baum Foundation the development of international research fellowship opportunities.

The need to increase research capacity and activity is a priority for our current President, Neena Modi, and the college staff are also rising to the challenge of ensuring all activity and outputs are evidence based. Political manifesto in all four countries of the UK, exerting political pressure including hosting debates and being the 'go to' organisation for advice on all child health issues, demands the college to be viewed as professional and well informed. Indeed many hours are spent working with the vast array of the UK wide government and arm's length bodies.

As the reach of the college and level of activity increases, there is a need to attract resources beyond those raised through membership or from restricted projects. In days of austerity, this is a real challenge that has led to the establishment of the Division of Business Development. As well as seeking unrestricted funds the divisions remit includes getting membership offers right, the delivery of interprofessional hot topic events and the running of the annual conference which now attracts over 2,000 paediatrician delegates and which is run in association with the Royal College of Nursing.

The college in 2017 celebrates its 21st birthday, and it is an incredible honour to be at the helm as we steer through the stormy water of the current NHS. The 160 current staff, based across the UK, are a highly motivated and committed team, and the college is a good place to work – we have just been named as one of the Sunday

Times top 100 employers. The dedication of the officers and members we work with is an inspiration to us all but of most importance to me as CEO is making sure the college provides the support required by all our members to improve child health in the UK and beyond.

The Devolved Nations and Republic of Ireland

24

Anna Murphy, John Morgan, Jo Sibert, John Jenkins, Moira Stewart, and Dennis Gill

The membership of the BPA and now college has always encompassed all parts of the United Kingdom as well as many paediatricians from the Republic of Ireland. Each country has had its own local mechanism of bringing paediatricians together as have many parts of England. The devolution of political powers to Scotland, Wales and Northern Ireland included health as one of the areas which was locally managed. This has led to increasing diversity in the way that paediatrics is delivered, and a four-nation approach has to be included in all that the college has done. Here we have reflections from the three devolved nations and Eire on the importance of the college.

History of the RCPCH in Scotland, Anna Murphy

In 1922, ten medical men in Edinburgh and Glasgow whose main interest was in diseases of children founded the Edinburgh and Glasgow Paediatric Club. The meetings were informal and friendly. In 1946 at the end of the Second World War, the name of the Club was changed to the Scottish Paediatric Society (SPS).

A. Murphy
Glasgow, UK

J. Morgan
Glamorgan, UK

J. Sibert (✉)
Cardiff, UK

J. Jenkins
Antrim, UK

M. Stewart
Belfast, UK

D. Gill
Dublin, Ireland

© Springer International Publishing Switzerland 2017
A. Craft, K. Dodd (eds.), *From an Association to a Royal College*,
DOI 10.1007/978-3-319-43582-4_24

The SPS and its meetings followed the same pattern as the Club, with most meetings being held in Aberdeen, Dundee, Edinburgh and Glasgow. The SPS continued to provide a unique and friendly forum for the exchange of information about the health and welfare of children. For both its Golden and Diamond Jubilee years, the society met with the British Paediatric Association in Aviemore.

Paediatricians in Scotland have had long associations with both the Royal College of Physicians and Surgeons in Glasgow (RCPSG) and the Royal College of Physicians in Edinburgh (RCPE). In the Edinburgh College a paediatrician has held a statutory position on the Council for many years, and, in more recent years, paediatricians Ian Laing and Morrice McCrae have served RCPE as Master of Music and College Historian, respectively. In Glasgow Professor James Hutchison, Professor of Child Health, was elected President of the College in 1968. The Paediatric Advisory Committee within the Glasgow College has had an important role in the organisation of symposia and examinations and giving advice to the college on child health matters.

In 1977 the paediatricians of the Glasgow College first discussed the proposal of the BPA to the setting up of a College of Paediatrics. The west of Scotland paediatricians of the time favoured the formation of a Faculty of Paediatrics within the Royal Colleges rather than a separate College of Paediatrics. Similarly in the east of the country, paediatricians who appreciated the support they received from RCPE preferred the idea of a faculty. The view of a number of paediatricians was that a new college could not hope to build up everything that the RCPE and the RCPSG had built up over the centuries. However there was concern in Scotland that the London Royal College of Physicians did not seem to be effective in representing the views of paediatricians and so, particularly in the east, paediatricians in time accepted that the way forward for child health was the setting up of a paediatric college. It was nearly 20 years before the proposal was discussed further, and it was in 1996 that the charter of the Royal College of Paediatrics and Child Health (RCPCH) was confirmed. In 1997 the Royal College of Physicians and Surgeons of Glasgow presented the new Royal College of Paediatrics and Child Health with a gavel and a desk lectern.

In 1998 Tom Turner was appointed the first RCPCH officer for Scotland. He set up the Scottish Committee. He was also Convenor of the Paediatric Advisory Committee of the Glasgow College and developed links from the outset between the new RCPCH and the Glasgow College. The issues discussed at the Scottish Committee were circulated to paediatricians throughout Scotland.

In 2001 Anna Murphy became officer for Scotland. With the advent of the Scottish Parliament and a Minister of Health who had stated that children were at the heart of his policies and priorities, an opportunity was seen to influence decision making on behalf of children and young people in Scotland. With support from Sir Alan Craft, RCPCH President, and Jo Sibert the officer for Wales, the RCPCH Scotland office was set up in 2001 in an annexe of the Royal College of Physicians in Queen Street, Edinburgh. The first office manager was Deanne Tomasino. The office was formally opened by the Princess Royal in November 2002 with Sir Alan Craft, in attendance.

In 2005 Adrian Margerison became Scottish officer, followed by Jim Beattie in 2008. The present Scottish officer is Peter Fowlie. Since the setting up of the RCPCH base in Scotland, the challenge has been to promote the partnership of the RCPCH, the ancient colleges, the SPS and more recently the Scottish Association of Community Child Health. The RCPCH office has had an important role in promoting this partnership and has worked closely with the Scottish Paediatric Society in organising the St Andrews Day Symposium each year. This event is hosted in alternate years in the Royal Colleges of Glasgow and Edinburgh, and an RCPCH office bearer gives the keynote lecture. A highlight of the 2007 Symposium was the attendance of the Princess Royal who gave the RCPCH address. The attendance at that Symposium was at its highest yet. When the Scottish Paediatric Society celebrated its 90th Anniversary Hilary Cass, RCPCH President gave the keynote address. RCPCH Scotland with the Scottish Paediatric Society contributed to the Annual RCPCH Meeting held in Glasgow in 2012. In the west the RCPSG Paediatric Advisory Committee is now synonymous with the RCPCH Regional Committee, and it is served by RCPCH administrative staff.

During the last 12 years, the Scottish RCPCH office has enabled effective communication and consultation with paediatricians working throughout the country. Three regional committees have been set up chaired by regional representatives. Formal and informal partnerships with the Scottish Government have been developed. Regular meetings with Ministers and the Chief Medical Officer take place, and Ministers attend RCPCH Policy Meetings at which topical child health issues are discussed. One example is that in conjunction with in conjunction with the Children and Families Department of the Scottish Government, RCPCH Scotland organises Fetal Alcohol Awareness sessions. Over 100 participants have attended these sessions including clinicians, social workers and Scottish Government staff.

A video-linked education lecture series was transmitted throughout Scotland over a 3-year period. Trainees now come for education days and whilst mother is being educated, she feeds her baby off camera!

Despite the strong loyalties towards the ancient colleges, it is evident that paediatricians working in Scotland today identify strongly with the RCPCH. The appointment of the officer for Scotland, the work of the Scottish Committee and the setting up of the RCPCH office in Scotland have all contributed to this.

History of the RCPCH in Wales, John Morgan and Jo Sibert

The coat of arms of the RCPCH shows as right supporter a figure representing Thomas Phaire in contemporary academic dress. He worked in West Wales, particularly Carmarthen and Cilgerran, as a doctor, lawyer, translator, poet and MP. He may rightly be considered the first paediatrician in Britain in that he published 'The Boke of Chyldren' in 1545. In this book he noted that the needs of children were different from adults. He emphasised the importance of the age of the child when symptoms started and the wisdom of simply waiting and observing the child. A commemorative plaque was erected in 1986 by the BPA, Welsh Paediatric Society (WPS), University of Wales College of Medicine and Welsh History of Medicine Society at St Llawddog's Church Cilgerran.

Paediatricians in Wales were strong supporters of the BPA with, Professor Arthur Goronwy Watkins (known as "Pop"), being Hon Treasurer 1958–1964 and president from 1966 to 1967. Paediatricians in Wales were also strong supporters of the formation of the RCPCH (donating the president's Giotto blue gown which has a red dragon embroidered on its collar); however, they also wished to maintain their links and functions as members of the WPS – Cymdeithas Pediatrig Cymru.

The WPS was formed in 1973 with the aims of advancing the study of paediatrics and child health in Wales and to foster friendship amongst paediatricians. Officers were democratically elected for fixed terms. They reported to and influenced developments in child health in Wales through the Welsh Standing Committee of the BPA, the Paediatric Sub-Committee of the Welsh Medical Committee and the Committee of the Welsh Paediatric Society. The biannual meetings, spring in the south and autumn in the north of Wales were well attended and of a good academic standard.

When the RCPCH was formed in 1996, the challenge was to preserve the functions of the WPS whilst supporting the RCPCH. The need for a Welsh identity for the Royal College became vital with the advent of devolution in Wales, following the referendum in 1997, and the establishment of the Welsh Assembly in 1999 if the needs of children were to be maintained. Representatives from Wales worked closely with those from Scotland (especially Dr Anna Murphy) and Northern Ireland in helping to achieve devolution in the college. This was helped very much by the presidents of the college especially Sir Alan Craft. The challenge of maintaining a presence for the RCPCH, whilst preserving the WPS has been achieved by having:

- The President of the WPS and the officer for Wales as the same person, elected through the RCPCH
- An office for the RCPCH in Wales
- Joint meetings twice a year
- A manager for the college in Wales
- An Annual St David's Lecture, in rotating venues throughout Wales
- A Welsh Committee for the college

In 1999, Dr John Morgan was appointed the first officer for Wales. He was already President of the WPS, and this joint role has continued since this time with Professor Jo Sibert (2002–2005), Dr Gwyneth Owen (2005–2008) and then Dr Iolo Doull. A separate RCPCH Council representative was reinstated initially Dr Duncan Cameron, followed by Iolo Doull, Justin Warner, Gwyneth Owen and Mair Parry. In 1997, the first office for the Royal College of Paediatrics and Child Health was established with the help of Catriona Williams (Chief Executive) at Children in Wales at 25

Windsor Place Cardiff. This was essentially just a desk, and we were very grateful for it; however, the need for a bigger office was clearly demonstrated.

So in 2004, we moved to Baltic House, Mount Stuart Square, Cardiff, in the Welsh Council for Voluntary Action building. The first manager for the RCPCH in Wales was Gwenda Page; she had a large part in facilitating the move. Some years later Gwenda moved to West Wales. The office in Baltic House was presented with a John Piper Lithograph, Nursery Frieze II, by the late Dr David Lewis a paediatrician from Aberystwyth and his wife Clarissa in 2007.

The meetings of the WPS have been a feature of paediatric life in Wales. The RCPCH in Wales has supported these meetings, and they are organised from the office in Baltic House. These meetings have continued to be very well attended and have a strong academic content in the presentations. The Annual WPS Lecture has attracted speakers from throughout the United Kingdom and Ireland; we have been fortunate to have all aspects of paediatrics and child health represented from neonatology through to community child health. The WPS has strong links with the Irish Paediatric Society, and we have had several joint meetings, which are remembered not only by the high standard of the presentations but also as marvellous social events.

When RCPCH Wales was established, a college lecture was also started: the St David's Lecture. This is now part of a meeting held as near as possible to St David's Day. The first lecture was given by Professor David P Davies in Cardiff, followed by Professor Jo Sibert in Swansea, and is now an annual event.

The office in Cardiff has enabled us to advance research concerning Child Health in Wales. Foremost amongst the projects is the Welsh Paediatric Surveillance Unit (WPSU). This is based on the British Paediatric Surveillance Unit (BPSU) where cards are sent out monthly asking consultants whether they have seen a number of rare conditions. We have concentrated in Wales on conditions too common for a BPSU study but too rare for study in a district. An example was serious child abuse, where the study provided important epidemiological evidence.

History of the RCPCH in Northern Ireland, John Jenkins and Moira Stewart

As part of the college response to the devolution of health across the UK, the RCPCH Ireland Committee was established in shadow form in 1999 with Professor Garth McClure as its first chair and had its first formal meeting the following year. The Ireland Committee differs from the Welsh and Scottish Committees, in that it seeks to represent paediatrics and child health across two separate countries, and therefore must take account of different jurisdictions, organisational structures for delivery of health and social care, training programmes (including examinations). Despite these differences, many RCPCH policy documents such as Facing the Future and training such as Child Protection, APLS, etc. are perceived as equally relevant to delivery of services in both Northern Ireland and the Republic of Ireland.

The Ireland Committee's terms of reference were to further the objects of the college and to represent the interests of members working in Northern Ireland and

Ireland and to fulfil the following functions and responsibilities in respect of both jurisdictions to:

(a) Represent and promote the interests of fellows and members of the college.
(b) Meet with CMO(s) for Ireland by arrangement.
(c) Respond to requests from the Irish departments for health.
(d) Facilitate paediatric examinations in Ireland.
(e) Build and maintain relationships with the University departments in Ireland and the Faculty of Paediatrics RCP Ireland.
(f) Report to RCPCH Council and the Faculty of Paediatrics RCP Ireland.
(g) Meet three times per year, once in Dublin, once at the RCPCH annual meeting and once in Belfast.

Its membership consisted of the chair (officer for Ireland), elected by the fellows and members throughout the island of Ireland and rotating between north and south, one or more senior officers of the RCPCH, together with representatives from Ireland and Northern Ireland. These include the regional representatives and regional advisors, together with those representing academic paediatrics, examinations and trainees in both jurisdictions.

In 2001 Dr John Jenkins became the first elected officer for Ireland. He was succeeded in 2004 by Professor Dennis Gill, then by Dr Moira Stewart from 2007 to 2012, and now by Dr Emma Curtis. During the first years of its existence, the Committee concentrated on the development of strategies for paediatric training, examinations, research and service provision for the whole island of Ireland and on increasing opportunities for cooperation in these areas between the two jurisdictions. A 3-year quality improvement project involved all the neonatal intensive care units throughout Ireland and Northern Ireland in association with the Vermont-Oxford Neonatal Network and EuroNeoNet. The Committee has continued to support multicentre research, most recently a follow-up twin study, and to hold joint meetings to discuss RCPCH initiatives such as Facing the Future and Service Frameworks.

Useful progress was also made with regard to linkages between training programmes in the UK and Ireland and between the paediatric examinations of RCPCH and RCPI, although difficulties remain in these areas. The removal of reciprocity of MRCPI for application to training programmes in the UK has had an impact on training experiences available to trainees and the opportunity for shared cross-border educational experiences. Dr Stewart currently undertakes the role of external assessor for penultimate year trainees in Ireland.

A further important aspect of the work of the Committee has been to help develop responses to a range of consultation documents relating to the future direction of paediatric and maternity services. There is evidence that this helped to raise the profile of the college as a body which can assist with development of policy initiatives in both the UK and Ireland. In January 2008 the Ireland Committee, in association with the Ulster Paediatric Society, organised a symposium entitled Priorities for Paediatrics and Child Health in Northern Ireland, with a keynote address by the Northern Ireland Chief Medical Officer Dr Michael McBride. This provided an important stimulus for the later development of a Framework for Children by the Northern Ireland Department of Health, Social Services and Public Safety.

In recent years significant progress has been made in the development of neonatal transport services both North and South of the border, and more recently a neonatal clinical network in Northern Ireland. However, despite these welcome developments, significant areas remain in both jurisdictions where services for children and young people require further development and resourcing. The current drive towards development of clinical networks is especially relevant to Northern Ireland, with its relatively small childhood population for whom subspecialty services can only be sustained in association with centres outside Northern Ireland, including those in Ireland. The priorities at this time for child health services in Ireland are to extend transport services, develop the new National Children's Hospital in Dublin and appraise options for delivery of specialist services for children with rare and complex conditions.

History of the RCPCH in Ireland, Dennis Gill

The Republic of Ireland (ROI) has a population of 4.5 million (approximately that of an NHS Health Region). ROI's 150 paediatricians are represented by the Faculty of Paediatrics RCPI. Northern Ireland (NI) has a population of 1.5 million. ROI training is similar to that in the UK and consists of basic specialist training of 2 years, followed by specialist registrar training of 5 years. ROI trainees take either MRCPI or MRCPCH, and many take both. There has been only a limited exchange of trainees between ROI and NOI.

In terms of governance, the RCPCH has regarded NI and ROI as single regions. The RCPCH has a regional adviser for NI and an officer for Ireland, who can come from either jurisdiction. The Ireland Committee embracing NI and ROI was established by Professor Sir Alan Craft in 1999. Its activities are well covered in the NI submission.

With regard to college examinations, the Part 1 examination has been purchased by RCPI from RCPCH. An Irish representative has sat on the Part 1 Board. The Part 2 RCPCH and RCPI examinations have always been separate, largely for medico-political and economic reasons. The RCPCH continues to provide external examiners for Part 2 MRCPI paediatrics.

RCPCH groups have come to Dublin for regional meetings, the British Association for Paediatric Nephrology in 2003 (hosted by Denis Gill), the British Paediatric Cardiologists in 2004 (hosted by Desmond Duff) and the British Society for Paediatric Endocrinology (hosted by Hilary Hoey).

The Annual RCPCH Conferences have always drawn a good attendance of Irish trainees and consultant paediatricians. Two proud 'paddy-atricians' (Denis Gill and Alf Nicholson) have won the Ulster Cup – the college's Golf Trophy, which was donated to the BPA in Newcastle, Co. Down by the Ulster paediatricians in 1936.

The Faculty of Paediatrics RCPI values greatly RCPCH documents, publications, reports, recommendations, many of which apply to Ireland as to the UK. The specialties of neonatology and cardiology in ROI have been recognised as part of the 'National Grid'. A good proportion of ROI paediatricians take the Archives of Disease in Childhood as their preferred paediatric publication.

NI and ROI, who play rugby as Ireland (United), were both very proud when Terence Stephenson was President of RCPCH (2009–2012). The Ireland Committee of the RCPCH has done much to bring us together. The BPSU has included ROI in its studies and mailings.

The island of Ireland, north and south, and its paediatricians have always had close connections with and commitment to the BPA/RCPCH. May it continue so.

Reflections of Members of Council

25

Geoff Lawson, Javed Iqbal, and Keith Dodd

Council was the governing body of the BPA and has similar authority in the College. The elected members of Council are trustees of the college and are elected on a regional basis, but as detailed in the governance section, this will soon change. Many of the College officers started their BPA/College careers as regional representatives.

They are drawn from a wide range of specialties, ranging from general paediatricians to tertiary specialists, both hospital and community based, and there are also representatives from paediatric specialties and academics.

The following accounts give a flavour of the experiences of paediatricians who have served on Council.

Geoff Lawson, Paediatrician, Sunderland

I qualified from Dundee in 1977 already knowing that I wanted to become a paediatrician. After my houseman's year, I did 12 months of adult medicine to help me through the first part MRCP multiple choice, which at that time was still an examination in adult medicine, without a paediatric option. The second part, slide show, written, oral and clinical examinations were paediatric, although examination fees

G. Lawson
Sunderland, UK

J. Iqbal
Burnley, UK

K. Dodd (✉)
Derby, UK

© Springer International Publishing Switzerland 2017
A. Craft, K. Dodd (eds.), *From an Association to a Royal College*,
DOI 10.1007/978-3-319-43582-4_25

still went to RCP. As I developed a political awareness, I became more and more disenchanted with our subsidiary role to a college of adult physicians and soon was a firm supporter of an independent college. Having become a consultant in Sunderland in 1991, I was too junior to have been intimately involved with this process which culminated in the formation of a Royal College in 1996, but was never in any doubt where my preference lay. Although this momentous event was the result of a gradual evolutionary process, I most clearly remember James Kempton, as the secretary of the BPA and then the RCPCH, going through detailed arrangements on gaining permission for Royal Assent and the formation of the new College's crest at open meetings at the BPA's AGM in York.

It followed that I was pleased to take the opportunity to put myself forward to become a regional representative to the College in 2003. An initiation session was offered at the college's first home in Hallam Street so that I was allowed to appreciate the vicarious liability that one accepted as an elected trustee of the College. Meetings which began at 10 am and finished at 4 pm were held in February, June and October. Initially I would catch an early (no, very early) train from Newcastle on the day of the meeting, but latterly found that my expenses were smaller and life more relaxed if I took an evening train the night before and stayed at the RCP in St. Andrews Place. It was not difficult to appreciate the historical backgrounds of the two colleges when staying in rooms dedicated to seventeenth-century physicians and founder members of RCP. It also made me realise that the twentieth century had been a period of significant change for RCP; in 1909, it had allowed ladies to be members for the first time and 87 years later had allowed paediatricians to become a distinct and separately governed organisation. So women came in and children went out.

During my elected time at the college, I became a part of the finance subgroup. We dealt with matters ranging from membership fees and expenses for examiners doing long-haul journeys to whether or not we should take over the vacated GMC building next door at Hallam Street or make a bold move and buy a much bigger building in Theobald's Road in Bloomsbury. Under the skillful guidance of Dr. Sue Hobbins and Mike Poole in retrospect, we seemed to have made reasonably prudent decisions.

In 2006, I was invited to celebrate our tenth birthday as a college at a dinner in London, which was attended by Anne Diamond. The following year I was interviewed for a newly created post of policy officer to support the Registrar Dr. Hilary Cass who shortly afterward left to take responsibility as head of school in Central London. As an officer I was given training in how best to relate to press enquiries, which helped enormously on the few occasions when this happened, and was frequently asked by David Ennis to draft college responses to documents issued by other organisations. Although exacting, this broadened my experience and enhanced my appreciation of the need for the College as an advocate for children in matters, ranging from how children who are political refugees should be treated to the paediatric training intentions of the RCGP.

In retrospect my closest involvement with a major strategic issue began with the policy conference in 2007. This began a process of forward planning of paediatric services led by Dr. Simon Lenton which was published in three consecutive years under the title *Modelling the Future*. I was asked to present an outline of the problems facing the delivery of care to acutely unwell children and subsequently chaired a small but well-informed group of wise paediatricians over 2 years. After a few face-to-face meetings and several iterations shared by email, we agreed on a report which became a central plank of 'Facing the Future' published in 2011.

My career as a clinical director in my Trust was undoubtedly enhanced by my more intimate involvement with the College. I feel as though I was able to contribute to College business, but was well aware of the important functions which the college sustained, often done quietly out of the glare of more public knowledge. Back in my day job, this awareness allowed me to prepare for changes whose embryonic form was being discussed.

As I travelled home on the 5 pm train from Kings Cross to Newcastle, I had time to collect my thoughts on the day's business and prepare feedback to colleagues 250 miles from the capital. Reaching home shortly before 9 pm, I would feel a little travel weary, but always felt that the opportunity to be involved with College business was a privilege and certainly not a burden. To have been part of the first years of our College's existence has been fulfilling. I would happily do it all again.

Dr. Javed Iqbal, Consultant Paediatrician, East Lancs Hospitals NHS Trust

Since the award of the Fellowship in 1997, I had served RCPCH in a variety of roles including tutor, host and examiner for clinicals, AAC member and a lead visiting assessor of hospital paediatric training. However, undoubtedly the most satisfying contribution has been as a Trustee and a member of RCPCH Council from 2008 to 2013. In this role I represented the north-west region of England, sat on the Finance Governance and Audit Committee (it later became the Finance and Corporate Services Committee) and the Budget Scrutiny Committee and chaired the Health and Safety Committee, as well as the Regional Committee for Higher Excellence Awards. I also represented the Council on the Paediatric Nephrology CSAC.

Over a period of 5 years, I had the fortune of contributing to discussions and decisions on a range of issues of great importance for the training of future paediatricians, paediatric clinical services in the UK as well as the governance of the College. I was able to bring my significant experience in Medical Education and Management here in the UK, as well as of working in a financially restricted environment abroad, before returning to my current consultant post. My training and experience, largely in the North West of England, conferred an understanding of the multicultural dynamics of health and disease in children.

Perhaps the most emotive contribution I have made in discussions within and outside the College Council has been around a belief that College and its members would benefit greatly by moving significant activity including the educational events to the regions. It has therefore been satisfying to see this happening increasingly in the recent years.

Professionally as my initial paediatric training took place in an excellent learning and working environment at Burnley in East Lancashire before spending a number of years at the Royal Manchester Children's Hospital, it has been particularly satisfying and a source of pride, serving East Lancashire, currently as clinical director of General Paediatrics and Lead for Clinical Education at the Family Care Division.

A Personal View: Keith Dodd

Two Flights from Scotland

Election to the Council of the BPA was a straightforward affair, a phone call one evening in 1988 from David Mellor, a paediatric neurologist in Nottingham who had just completed his term of office on Council. He asked if I wished to be nominated to succeed him – after all, he said, it was the turn of a DGH paediatrician. That was it.

So began my involvement with the BPA/college which would span the next three decades and 22 years on Council.

I had been appointed as a consultant in Derby after training in paediatrics in Bury St. Edmunds, Liverpool and Glasgow; my enthusiasm fired as a student at UCH by Leonard Strang's team, including Colin Normand, Osmond Reynolds, Max Friedman, Geoffrey Hatcher and Charles Dent. I was not alone; eight in my year went into paediatrics.

Advised by John Hay, head of department in Liverpool, who was at the time president of the BPA, I took the adult membership exam, in common with the majority of paediatric trainees those days. My time as a registrar in adult medicine was a chore but with hindsight invaluable, and I was left with a strong sense of allegiance to the London RCP, reinforced by having to host their exam for the first time in Croydon before returning to paediatric training, this time in Glasgow.

My early years as a new consultant in Derby were a baptism of fire. My colleague Tim Chambers' move to Bristol was followed by Leonard Arthur's trial for attempted murder (q.v. Chap. 14, Ethics) and untimely death, leaving me as senior in a department whose Children's Hospital was threatened with closure and relocation to a couple of vacated obstetric wards. Overcoming these challenges taught me a lot about medical politics, and I was pleased to take up the offer of a post on BPA Council.

But my gentle introduction to Council was soon to be shattered. The equivocal result of the 1987 BPA referendum, showing equal support for a faculty on the one hand and for an independent college on the other, was followed by a proposal for an interdependent college with the three UK Royal Colleges of Physicians. Returning from a meeting in Edinburgh by plane, June Lloyd and Tim Chambers, respectively, president and hon. sec. of the BPA, were minded, as they flew over Derby, to suggest I be given the task of preparing a draft charter on behalf of the BPA.

Drawing up an interdependent charter was hard work, great fun, but clearly a lost cause. None of the three ancient colleges wanted it; they preferred us to be a faculty.

Nor did most paediatricians, as was confirmed at the next referendum in 1990, which threw it out. I sometimes wonder if June Lloyd, a strong advocate of an independent college, had seized the opportunity to demonstrate that a closer working relationship with the ancient colleges was unworkable, by pursuing the cause of an interdependent college. If so it was a political master stroke.

The views of paediatricians hardened after this, the final referendum just 2 years later confirming strong support for an independent college.

Personally, my own allegiance to the London RCP and the BPA diminished as I learned at first hand of the difficulties successive BPA presidents, John Forfar, June Lloyd and David Hull, had experienced gaining our own voice for paediatrics and in working with three separate colleges of physicians. (However the experience would later be put to good use when preparing the College Charter.)

Roy Meadow's account of the subsequent battle for our college (Chap. 1) accurately records the huge task he faced on taking office. June Lloyd and David Hull had laid the groundwork, but a host of others outside our specialty needed to be persuaded to accept the case for a Charter for a college of paediatrics.

In his year as president-elect, Roy sat as an observer on the major committees of the BPA, apparently asleep, raising an eyebrow occasionally, commenting rarely and taking no notes. I was worried.

But my concerns were unfounded. Roy Meadow had waited over 20 years for this moment, and when the time came, he hit the ground running. He confronted the opposition, rallied support at home and abroad with a torrent of letters and united the BPA membership in a whirlwind campaign lasting the best part of 2 years.

His account of the receipt of the letter from the Privy Council supporting our case omits one important detail. He initially told us, brow wrinkled and apparently furious, that our case had been rejected by the Privy Council. Then out came the champagne.

The next 2 years were a blur, with events tumbling over each other. Visits to the Privy Council at Downing St. and to Buckingham Palace to meet our new Patron, the Princess Royal, are recalled in James Kempton's narrative (Chap. 20), culminating in the inaugural meeting in York in Spring 1997 and the commemorative service in the Minster masterminded by David Baum, where I also noted the sight of trainees from a wide range of ethnic and religious backgrounds seated side by side on a pew opposite. Wonderful.

On a personal level, these were the busiest years of my life: the purpose-built new Derbyshire Children's Hospital opened in 1996, bringing together all children's services on one site, and an academic department of paediatrics followed soon after. At home, our four children successfully moved away to university and to nursing, while my wife Jenny was studying for her degree in Fine Arts.

The new college got off to a flying start, the adoption of its new responsibilities proceeding remarkably smoothly. The untimely sudden death of our second President David Baum on a fund-raising bike ride was a tragic loss. He had energised the college with his rare combination of academic, political and personal skills, and he would have achieved so much more.

After a 5-year term as honorary secretary of the BPA/RCPCH, I was elected officer for health services, with roles on a wide range of national committees and bodies, reflecting the recognition and status of the new college. We were successful in lobbying for Children's Commissioners in each of the four nations and a National Service Framework for Children. But sadly we did not persuade the government immediately of the need for a minister for children.

One of my most pleasant tasks was to liaise with the three Scottish Royal Colleges, which involved regular visits to Edinburgh and Glasgow to attend a Joint Paediatric Committee, of which June Lloyd had once commented 'this committee will take some time to bed down'. By now it was running smoothly and I always enjoyed the visits to my old training ground and home. Flying back one evening over the Lake District Mountains, I could clearly see the high-level route leading to Pillar Rock outlined by the setting sun, an exhilarating prospect for a keen fell-walker.

After 17 years, it was time to return to the hills.

Academy of Medical Royal Colleges (AoMRC)

26

Alan Craft

One of the benefits of being a royal college is that we are able to take our place amongst the other colleges. The presidents meet together at the Academy of Medical Royal Colleges.

At the time of the First World War, there were colleges of physicians and surgeons in Edinburgh, Dublin and London, while Glasgow had a single faculty of physicians and surgeons. Proposals in the 1920s for a union between physicians and surgeons in London did not come to fruition. The obstetricians formed their college in 1929 and received their Royal Charter in 1947.

Since then a number of new faculties and colleges have developed, and as a result, there is considerable variation between specialties, which may be represented by different bodies in different areas. The general practitioners formed their college in 1952. Members of some specialties, e.g. pathologists and radiologists, formed new colleges of their own in the 1970s. Psychiatrists progressed through the Association of Medical Officers of Lunatic Asylums (1841), the Medico-Psychological Association (1856) and the Royal Medico-Psychological Association (1926) to a college in 1971. More recently the anaesthetists, formerly a faculty of the College of Surgeons, and the ophthalmologists have formed their own colleges. Specialists in Public Health Medicine formed a faculty between the colleges of physicians. The Royal College of Paediatrics and Child Health was established in 1996, and the College of Emergency Medicine became a college in its own right in 2008.

A. Craft
Newcastle, UK

© Springer International Publishing Switzerland 2017
A. Craft, K. Dodd (eds.), *From an Association to a Royal College*,
DOI 10.1007/978-3-319-43582-4_26

Dates of College Charters

Royal College of Surgeons of Edinburgh 1505
Royal College of Physicians of London 1518
Royal College of Physicians and Surgeons of Glasgow (Faculty, 1599) 1962
Royal College of Physicians of Ireland 1654
Royal College of Physicians of Edinburgh 1681
Royal College of Surgeons of Ireland 1784
Royal College of Surgeons of England 1800
Royal College of Obstetricians and Gynaecologists 1929
(Royal Charter 1947)
Faculty of Dental Surgery 1947
Royal College of General Practitioners (Royal Charter, 1967) 1952
Royal College of Pathologists (College, 1963) 1970
Royal College of Psychiatrists (Society, 1841) 1971
Royal College of Radiologists (Faculty, 1939) 1975
Faculty of Public Health Medicine 1978
Faculty of Occupational Medicine 1978
Royal College of Anaesthetists (Faculty 1948, Royal Charter 1992) 1988
Royal College of Ophthalmologists (Society, 1880) 1988
Faculty of Pharmaceutical Medicine 1989
Royal College of Paediatrics and Child Health 1996
Royal College of Emergency Medicine 2008

In 1976, a Conference of Medical Royal Colleges and Faculties was formed. The need for a body such as the Conference followed the formation of the increasing number of colleges and faculties as shown above, not only to consider Joint Consultative Committee (JCC) business but also to promote the aim of jointly preserving standards in the best interests of medicine. The JCC was a joint committee between the BMA and representatives of the colleges. This Conference had 16 members (two from each of the major colleges and one from each of the others, including the Scottish but not the Irish college).

Until 1988, the Conference met only quarterly on the day before JCC and always in London. At that time it became apparent that additional meetings, the agenda for which was not circumscribed by JCC matters, were necessary if the Conference was to maintain its voice on standards. This was seen to require a facility to receive reports from subcommittees and working parties, while taking into account the responsibilities and powers of individual colleges and reducing the possibility that the position of colleges might be weakened by their own increasing numbers.

In 1991, the Conference set up a working party to investigate its future requirements, in terms of function, structure, name and secretarial support. There was a widespread recognition that the Conference was increasingly important in assisting medical royal colleges to establish and maintain high standards of patient care, through training and monitoring performance. The demands on the chairman of Conference increased considerably, and it became impossible to be properly supported by the staff of one college alone.

It was therefore agreed that from January 1993, a Conference office, staffed by an executive secretary, should be established in support of the Conference, especially the chairman and honorary secretary. A further member of staff was recruited in 1995.

In February 1996, it was agreed to invite the presidents of the Royal College of Physicians of Ireland and the Royal College of Surgeons in Ireland to become full members of the Conference of Medical Royal Colleges.

In April 1996, the Conference of Medical Royal Colleges agreed to change its name to Academy of Medical Royal Colleges and charitable status was granted in July.

In December 1996, the Royal College of Paediatrics and Child Health was elected as a full member and the College of Emergency Medicine became a member in 2008.

Over time the Academy established a series of committees, generally comprising representatives from all member colleges to oversee and direct its work. The focus of the Academy's work is around medical education and, increasingly, standards of clinical care. A major review of the Academy's governance was undertaken in 2009/2010. Following the approval of the Charity Commission, this resulted in the establishment of a board of trustees, which includes independently appointed members, to be responsible for the governance of the organisation separate from the council of Academy members which would be responsible for healthcare policy and professional issues.

In January 2011, the Academy realised a long-term goal of moving into its own property. The Academy office is at 10 Dallington Street, London, EC1. The property has its own meeting rooms, so, importantly, the Academy can now host all its meetings on its own premises. Two RCPCH presidents have been elected as chairman of the AoMRC, Alan Craft and Terence Stephenson. The current chairman is Dame Sue Bailey, a forensic child psychiatrist and Hon FRCPCH.

Is the Academy effective? The major objection of the RCPL to the formation of the RCPCH was that "Balkanisation" with a proliferation of colleges would dilute and weaken the colleges' traditional influence with government. Although the Academy is ostensibly a single voice on occasions, individual colleges have been "picked off." This was evident in the very acrimonious debates around the Lansley reforms of the NHS where an initial united approach of major opposition of the colleges was eroded by political pressure. However, more recently, it was the Academy who brokered an agreement between the government and the BMA over the junior doctors' dispute. The Academy is a powerful body when each college is prepared to subjugate its own sovereignty to a collective will. Not surprisingly this does not always happen. In an increasingly politicised NHS, it is essential that the royal colleges speak with one voice.

Conspectus

27

Alan Craft, Keith Dodd and Judith Ellis

The starting point for this history posed the question: was the struggle to become a separate college worth it?
  Here Chief Executive Judith Ellis and the joint editors of this volume reflect on this.

The college is in a strong position to continue *leading the way in children's health*. The Royal College of Paediatrics and Child Health in its 21st year has 17,000 members. It continues to provide educational and professional support to all these members, which each year includes around 3,000 doctors in training, forever expanding its educational, conference and event activity. This activity now attracts wider child health professionals with some just attending events or signing on to Paediatric Care Online, but others joining as affiliate members. The college is increasingly producing educational material for direct access by children, young people and their families, for example, medicines for children leaflets; MindEd, which is a modular educational package around mental health; and disability matters. It has become the 'go to' organisation for advice around child health for politicians and senior health officials in the UK and beyond, including facilitating access to the child and young person's voice. The colleges & Us virtual network and engagement collaborative is being increasingly used by other colleges and organisations to access the CYP voice and to make sure all consultations have that CYP focus. Over 200 members have received media training and the college provides on average 20 press briefings each week on a diverse range of topics. All media and policy output are based on the highest available level of evidence and the

A. Craft
Newcastle, UK

K. Dodd
Derby, UK

J. Ellis (✉)
London, UK

© Springer International Publishing Switzerland 2017
A. Craft, K. Dodd (eds.), *From an Association to a Royal College*,
DOI 10.1007/978-3-319-43582-4_27

RCPCH supports the development of nationwide guidance (e.g. over 200 NICE and SIGN guidelines). The Facing the Future suite of standards are forever increasing which, with the reliable workforce census data gathered each 2 years, is helping members and the NHS to better workforce plan and commission. The college is using these standards to inform around 25 invited reviews of paediatric services each year and hosts three government-funded audits (e.g. neonatal, diabetes and epilepsy care). Its relationship with paediatric specialist groups in the UK and further afield is ever improving. The sharing of expertise has led to an increase of global activity, with an income of around £1 million for this.

How Has the RCPCH Made a Difference?

In his critical commentary on the formation of the college in Chap. 2 of this book, Tim Chambers lists the college's successes and missed opportunities as he sees them. While it is impossible to judge what the BPA alone could have achieved, his assessment is generally fair, and the achievements he lists are impressive.

However, most paediatricians who worked through this period of rapid change in health service provision would view the college's successes even more positively.

The College got off to a cracking start, with an impressive succession of beknighted presidents and the elevation of June Lloyd, a key founder, to the House of Lords. Unfortunately June Lloyd was never able to have the influence that she undoubtedly would have done as she had a major stroke soon after her ennoblement.

The acceptance by the other medical royal college was warm, generous and immediate and considerably enhanced by a pleasantly informal president's dinner and evening entertainment hosted by David Baum with the accompaniment of kazoos and a visit to Ronnie Scott's.

Perhaps the most important reflection of the college's influence has been in achieving a single professional voice for child health and for paediatricians, supplanting the separate roles of the three ancient colleges of physicians. This is not only evident in the media but also in the regard in which the colleges is held among the other colleges, the Academy of Medical Royal Colleges and the Department of Health. Influential as it was, We doubt anyone would accept that the BPA, or a Paediatric Faculty of the RCP (London), could have commanded this influence and respect.

The college has overseen a period of dramatic consultant expansion which has been achieved through major transformation of the training programmes and the examinations, both areas over which the BPA had little influence.

Moreover it is fulfilling its primary aim of improving children's health, both through advocacy and more recently by actively involving children, young people and families in the core of its work.

Dr Sheila Shribman, when reflecting on her time at the DH, said 'We now need to stop talking to ourselves and talk to all of the others who need to be interested in children'. This relates particularly to the increasing recognition of the importance of the challenges of transition to adult services. This has meant us re-establishing links with the RCPs and working together in partnership for the benefit of patients.

The work of the research division affords several examples of the college's enhanced influence, not least through the work of the BPSU, now a model adopted internationally. The division's early commitment to health service research, including the regular workforce census and modelling, led to several influential reports on workforce planning and service configuration which are gradually gaining acceptance and being implemented nationally. Similarly the work in developing paediatric formulary medicines for children is seen to be of international importance.

The concerns about the effects of Balkanisation and the loss of influence were evident long before the RCPCH came into being. We were the latest in a long line of other disciplines which had obtained autonomy from their original parent colleges. There does now seem an inevitability to the formation of the college, and in our view, we have made a pretty good job of becoming an influential voice for children and their health.

Clearly there is much more to be done, not least in tackling inequalities, obesity and child and adolescent mental health and in securing a fairer allocation of resources for children, but the college is well positioned to take on these challenges.

We look forward to the next 12 years when we will reach our centenary and hope that this volume will provide a platform for future paediatricians to chronicle our further development.

Appendix

We include here an extract from the third volume of the history of the BPA 1928–1988, edited by Forfar, Jackson and Laurance.

Extracts from the Third Volume of the BPA History

John Forfar, Anthony Jackson and Bernard Laurance

'The longer you can look back, the further you can look forward', Sir Winston Churchill reminded the Royal College of Physicians of London in 1944.

In the nineteenth century, the birth rate in Britain was about three times as high as it is now. In the early Victorian era, children were plentiful, so plentiful that there were those who considered them expendable.

Children were exploited on the land, down the mines and in the factories which exemplified the Industrial Revolution. They were paid a pittance and were small, small enough to creep as oilers and cleaners under the new machinery responsible for creating Britain's rising prosperity or to crawl up chimneys where their size made them much more effective chimney sweeps than their adult masters. Most Victorian families were large enough to sustain the culling which death from disease, poverty and social neglect imposed upon them. One child in five was dead by the age of 5 years and childhood disease crippled many others. During the century, however, a changing sense of human values was altering these attitudes. Writers such as Charles Dickens were contributing to the awakening of a new social conscience. He advocated the establishment of children's hospitals. Others, including doctors such as Doctor Barnardo, were opening homes for deprived children. There was concern when recruitment for the Boer War revealed that a high proportion of young men were unfit for service due to the effects of childhood disease. War, that hothouse of technological and social change, was playing its part in promoting better appreciation of the rights and needs of children.

In the changing social climate of the twentieth century, there were greater opportunities for moving up the social scale and into more remunerative employment. Given improved education and opportunity, parents' social aspirations for their children increased. But the education and support available for a child often depended

© Springer International Publishing Switzerland 2016   211
A. Craft, K. Dodd (eds.), *From an Association to a Royal College*,
DOI 10.1007/978-3-319-43582-4

on the number of other children in the family, and this was an incentive to reduce family size. As the birth rate fell, children became scarcer and, to put the matter at its lowest economic level, each became more valuable. The era in which children 'should be seen and not heard' had passed; they were now beginning to be heralded as 'the seed corn of the nation'. Paralleling these changed attitudes were new expectations of parents that such children as they had should be born healthy and remain so. The aim of medicine, particularly among doctors concerned with children, was to achieve this objective. Thus, in 1928, there was formed in Britain an association of doctors dedicated to the improvement of children's health and welfare.

Objectives and Philosophy

The British Paediatric Association or 'BPA' can now look back 60 years. Its first objectives as stated by its founders were clear and simple: 'The advancement of the study of paediatrics and the promotion of friendship among paediatricians'. These are still among the objectives although no longer officially so recorded. In keeping with the BPA's transformation from its early position as a club to its present status as a national professional association and registered charity, there is now no reference to social relationships among paediatricians. The objectives as defined in the members' handbook now recognise wider and more clearly defined professional responsibilities. '... The Association is established to advance, for the benefit of the public, education in child health and paediatrics and to relieve sickness by promoting the improvement in paediatric practice. In furtherance of the above object...the Association shall have the following powers:

(a) To promote paediatric research and to publish the results of such research
(b) To organise scientific meetings
(c) To advise government and other professional bodies on problems of child health
(d) To do all such other lawful things as shall further the above objects'

Recently (1985) these objectives were further expanded as follows:

(a) To provide authoritative views on childhood diseases
(b) To promote child health
(c) To develop and promote good practice in the care of the sick, handicapped, deprived or disadvantaged child
(d) To promote scientific research into the causes, prevention and treatment of childhood diseases
(e) To disseminate the results of research through scientific meetings and the *Archives of Disease in Childhood*, the official journal of the Association
(f) To act as a national advisory body on all aspects of the health of children and adolescents to the government, the professions and voluntary and statutory bodies
(g) To provide a national platform for paediatrics and child health

(h) To provide representatives for international, national and local statutory and non-statutory committees dealing with child health and childhood disease

(i) To maintain an interest in and advise upon undergraduate, postgraduate and continuing professional medical education in paediatrics and child health

(j) To foster good relations between British paediatricians and paediatricians in European and other overseas countries, including developing countries

Dr Hector Cameron (1878–1958), the first paediatrician to Guy's Hospital and writer of the first history of the BPA [1], considered that paediatricians were exceptional in their friendliness and lack of worldly rivalry and attributed this to 'the lack of mercenary considerations that sometimes beguile our surgical and gynaecological colleagues especially'. Perhaps personal attributes determine the professional calling which paediatricians have chosen to follow. Young children know no social distinctions.

A History of the British Paediatric Association

As a former President of the Association said, when contrasting the different attitudes and demeanour of physicians for adults with those of paediatricians, 'Can you imagine the formalised bedside manner of the consultant physician for adults allowing him to sit on the floor to talk to a toddler?' As Cameron commented, 'rivalry there is among paediatricians, not in the mercenary sphere but rather in the field of academic achievement and in providing the best possible service for children and their parents'.

The aim 'to advise government and other professional bodies' has involved no party politics. Indeed, the role of the BPA has often been to try to prevent the vagaries of doctrinaire party politics and polarised political philosophies from disturbing the continuous evolution of a child health service suitable for the children of this country and to guide the political machinery towards priorities determined only by the true needs of child health without considerations of political popularity. The care of children should be independent of the complexion of the government of the day and of political expediency.

While the BPA is concerned primarily with the cure and alleviation of childhood disease and the promotion of child health, its remit extends beyond any narrow concept of childhood health. It includes, for instance, such social problems as child abuse, increasing violence and crime, problems which affect children and at the same time have part of their origins in childhood upbringing and experience. The BPA seeks to alert government, other bodies and individuals concerned with the welfare of children to practices and environmental conditions it considers inimical to the mental, emotional and physical well-being of children. It has made representations about problems such as the content of television programmes and videos, social and sex education in schools, the problems of adolescence and the manner in which handicapped children are further disadvantaged by many current administrative practices and organisational arrangements which relate to the past but fail to meet the needs of the present.

In 1988, the BPA has over 2000 members. The range of its activities is now wide, and it recognises few limits to the scope of its involvement in childhood problems. This book is a short history of the BPA published to mark its Diamond Jubilee: it summarises the broad range of the Association's activities and development over the last 60 years.

References

1. Cameron HC. The British Paediatric Association 1928–1952. London: The British Paediatric Association; 1955.

The Early History of the BPA

The history of the first 25 years of the British Paediatric Association (1928–1952) written by Hector Cameron was followed by another history covering the next 16 years [1] (1952–1968) written by Professor Victor Neale (1899–1970), first Professor of Paediatrics in Bristol. This chapter summarises and complements these two volumes. Quotations are from one or the other of these two histories unless otherwise stated.

The Development of Paediatrics as a Separate Discipline in Britain

The BPA can reasonably claim to have established paediatrics as an identifiable organised medical discipline in Britain. In earlier times, there were, of course, doctors who interested themselves particularly in children, but they did so in an individualistic isolated way. Two of the earliest British pioneers whom history records as paediatric innovators and whose achievements are so recognised by paediatric associations in Britain and in the United States were Thomas Phaer (1510–1560) and George Armstrong (1719–1789).

As far as is known, Thomas Phaer wrote the first British textbook of paediatrics, 'The Boke of Chyldren', published in 1544. It contained 20,000 words, one hundredth the length of a comprehensive British paediatric textbook of today. Although not a Welshman, Thomas Phaer lived and worked in Cilgerran in the old county of Pembroke. He was not only a physician of children. Such were the limitations of paediatric knowledge in the sixteenth century and the breadth of Phaer's erudition that in addition to ministering to the health of children, he was also a lawyer, writer of a textbook on law, Member of Parliament, poet and translator of the classics. Further, he was Customs Officer for the ports of South West Wales, an appointment which led to him being threatened with hanging by some of the smuggling fraternity who objected to the assiduous manner in which he performed his duties. Thomas Phaer's book was reprinted in 1955 [2] on the initiative of Victor Neale and Dr Hugh

Wallis (1914–1963) (Bath), both past members of the BPA. In 1986 the BPA was pleased to be associated with the dedication of a memorial tablet to Thomas Phaer in Saint Llawddog's Church in Cilgerran (Plate 46).

George Armstrong (1719–1789) was a Scotsman who emigrated to London [3]. The Ambulatory Paediatric Association of America accepts him as the Father of Ambulatory Paediatrics. He limited his practice to the care of children, introduced the concept of teaching mothers about preventive health measures during acute illness visits and established a Dispensary for the Infant Poor in London in 1767. He also wrote a paediatric textbook entitled 'An Essay on the Diseases Most Fatal to Infants' [4]. It was nearly two centuries later, however, before paediatrics as such was recognised.

Paediatrics has developed in different ways in different countries. Whereas in the rest of Europe and the United States doctors trained as paediatricians frequently work as primary care physicians of children, in Great Britain the primary care of patients of all ages has always been the responsibility of general practitioners – whose training in paediatrics until recently was often seriously deficient – and secondary (specialist) care has been the responsibility of consultants.

Before the National Health Service (NHS), consultants gave their services to hospitals in an honorary capacity, their income being derived from private practice. Although in the 1920s and 1930s they earned an ample income from the rich in order to work unpaid among the poor, their status would not have led the German surgeon Von Bergmann to write as he did of London surgeons in the Victorian era, expressing 'his utter amazement at their fine houses, lavish hospitality and worldly superfluity'.

Young parenthood, however, tends to be an impecunious period of life, so children have always been a very small part of private practice and private paediatric practice in the 1920s and 1930s which was so financially unrewarding and attracted only the most dedicated. Cameron claimed in 1920 that he was the first physician to relinquish his appointment as a physician of adults at his teaching hospital (Guy's) in order to devote his time wholly to the care of sick children. Thus in 1928 there were very few paediatricians working solely with children; the care of children in hospital and the teaching of paediatrics at the time the BPA was founded were largely undertaken by a few interested general physicians whose work was mainly with adults.

As a consequence of this system of staffing, Britain lagged behind the United States and some other European countries in the development of paediatrics and of a body of doctors who specialised in children's diseases. In 1929, when the BPA could muster fewer than 60 members, nearly all of whom also practised adult medicine, it was estimated that 1300 physicians in the United States confined their practice to children.

While physicians of adults had some knowledge of the illnesses of older children, many had little, or none, of the illnesses of infants. One of the first three Honorary Members of the BPA, Sir Thomas Barlow (1845–1945) (Great Ormond Street [GOS]* and University College Hospital, London), was an exception. He first described infantile scurvy which became known as Barlow's disease. Both Dr John

Thomson (1856–1926) in Edinburgh and Dr (later Professor Sir Frederic) Still (1868–1941) (GOS and King's College Hospital) in London practised solely among, and taught about, sick children from the first rather than transferring their interest from adults to children as Cameron did. Thomson and Still are therefore regarded as the 'Fathers' of British Paediatrics.

The BPA Forerunners

Society for the Study of Children's Disease

Physicians interested in children rarely met for discussion until the Society for the Study of Children's Disease was founded in London in 1900. In comparison with the ill-attended inaugural meeting of The Hospital for Sick Children, Great Ormond Street, London, will henceforth be referred to as 'GOS'.

BPA 28 years later this Society began with a flourish. There were more than 80 original members drawn from all parts of Britain including Scotland and Northern Ireland and in addition to a Chairman, two Honorary Secretaries and an Honorary Treasurer, a Council of 22 members was elected. The Society included many who later achieved great distinction such as Dr (later Sir) Humphrey Rolleston (1862–1944) and Dr Parkes Weber (1863–1962), physicians; Mr (later Sir) Robert Jones (1858–1933), orthopaedic surgeon; and Mr (later Sir) Harold Stiles (1863–1946), plastic surgeon. Meetings were mostly clinical. Cases were demonstrated and eagerly discussed (the rarer the case, the better), and such 'giants' as Rolleston (who later became an original Honorary Member of the BPA) and Parkes Weber would vie with each other in vigorous clinical discussion. Parkes Weber continued to attend clinical meetings until shortly before his death at the age of 99 years, and current older members of the BPA may recall proudly presenting a 'first' case of some rare disease at the Royal Society of Medicine only to be discomfited by Parkes Weber describing in remarkable detail several cases of the same condition. The auspicious inauguration and early promise of the Society for the Study of Children's Diseases appear to have been followed later by unrecorded decline and disappearance.

The Children's Clinical Club

There was also in London at this time the Children's Clinical Club, a select group of a dozen or so consultants who met in each other's houses. Still was the first secretary. Thomson was an active member and travelled from Edinburgh to attend meetings. Cameron, Still and Thomson, the 'full-time' paediatricians, along with adult physicians who also practised paediatrics such as Sir Robert Hutchison (1872–1960) (GOS and the London Hospital), attended regularly, while others such as Sir William Osler (1849–1919) from Oxford and Dr (later Professor) Leonard Findlay (1878–1947) from Glasgow attended occasionally. Hutchison, a tall lean figure in grey morning dress, provided much of the wit and wisdom at the Clinical Club meetings. Although he lived to the age of 88 and was to take on the duties of

President (1938–1941) of the Royal College of Physicians of London at 66, he wrote at 55 to congratulate his young recently appointed assistant, Dr Bernard Schlesinger (1896–1984) (GOS and University College Hospital), 'As I get old and sour and lazy I want a young genial and energetic junior first to make people glad when I take long holidays'. The dominant force in the Children's Clinical Club, however, despite the distance which he had to travel, was Thomson. Such was his influence that the club's demise followed shortly after his own. Author of the leading paediatric textbook of the day, he died 2 years before the BPA was established. When a memorial tablet to him was unveiled in the Royal Hospital for Sick Children in Edinburgh in 1929, Barlow, Still and Hutchison were all present and gave eloquent appreciative addresses.

The Preposterous Club

With the decline of the two earlier societies, a club formed by a more vigorous group of enthusiasts began to flourish. Cameron and Dr David Forsyth (1877–1941) (London) started a dining group named the Preposterous Club with the aim of fostering cooperation between those involved in 'pre-' and 'post-'natal care. Sir Eardley Holland (1879–1967), Honorary Member of the BPA and President of the Royal College of Obstetricians and Gynaecologists, was a member: Medical Officers of Health and administrators from the recently formed Ministry of Health were also members. Not until 1979 was such a varied membership, embracing most branches of child health, again achieved – by the BPA. The Preposterous Club turned interest away from paediatric rarities to a study of commoner childhood problems. Dr Harold Waller (1881–1955) (Mother and Babies Hospital, Woolwich), whose studies of breastfeeding are classic, was a prominent representative of doctors working in Infant Welfare Clinics. Such was his persuasiveness that more than 80 % of the mothers at Woolwich were breastfeeding at a time when 30 % or so was all that could be achieved at most other hospitals. When asked how he had persuaded the midwives to renounce bottle feeding, in such vogue at the time, he replied quietly 'in many cases I have had to outlive them'. Later, as Cameron wrote, somewhat sadly, 'Forsyth had the misfortune to be so overcome by the persuasive force of Freud's teaching that finally, to his undoing, it possessed him to the exclusion of all other interests'. To those who have read Cameron's sensitive book about disturbed behaviour in children, 'The Nervous Child' [5], this seems a somewhat paradoxical comment.

The Edinburgh and Glasgow Paediatric Club: Scottish Paediatric Society

In Scotland, the Edinburgh and Glasgow Paediatric Club was formed in 1922. Patients were demonstrated at twice yearly meetings following which 'the members dined together in amity'. Thomson was the first Chairman, and Findlay, later Professor of Medical Diseases of Children in the University of Glasgow, was the first Secretary, and there were ten other members. Two members from Newcastle, one of them Dr (later Professor Sir James) Spence (1892–1954), were elected in 1924. In 1947, the club was reconstituted as the Scottish Paediatric Society with Professor Geoffrey Fleming (1882–1952) of Glasgow as the first President.

The Provincial Children's Club

The Provincial Children's Club was formed about 1924 but seems to have been so informal that no minutes were kept. Meetings were at convenient hotels in Liverpool (Professor Norman Capon, 1892–1975, and Dr Dingwall Fordyce, 1875–1940), Manchester (Drs Charles Lapage, 1879–1947; J F Ward, 1887–1950; and H T Ashby, 1880–1952), Birmingham (Sir Leonard Parsons, 1879–1950, and Professor James Smellie, 1894–1961) or Leeds (Professor Wilfred Vining, 1883–1967). All the Provincial Club members were later to become founding members of the BPA.

The Founding of the British Paediatric Association

Dr Donald Paterson (1890–1969) (Westminster and GOS), a Canadian of Scottish extraction who had qualified in medicine in Edinburgh, was the driving force in the establishment of the BPA. He was a handsome, immaculately dressed, kindly outspoken extrovert who did not hesitate to ruffle the feathers of senior colleagues in advancing new ideas for promoting the interests of paediatrics. He had persuaded Still of the need for an Association and to become the first President (Plate 1). Still was the natural choice as he was universally regarded as the leader of the little band of children's physicians. The inaugural meeting was held on 2nd February 1928 in Still's House at 28 Queen Anne Street, London. Despite invitations to twenty-four, only six attended: Still, Paterson, Drs Hugh Thursfield (1869–1944) (GOS), Frederick Poynton (1869–1943) (Middlesex Hospital), Morley Fletcher (1864–1950) (St Bartholomew's Hospital) and R C Jewesbury (1878–1971) (St Thomas's Hospital).

The first problem encountered was the title of the Association and the use of the word 'paediatric', a word hardly used in Great Britain until then and one of which Still was not enamoured. 'Paediatrics' is derived from the Greek words for a child (*pais*) and for a doctor (*iatros*). The Americans, who had been using the word for some time, spelt it without the 'a' causing confusion with words derived from the Latin pes (a foot). Before the meaning of the word 'paediatrics' was better understood, some early paediatricians found themselves confronted by corpulent men with flat feet or elderly ladies with hallux valgus. When Dr Hugh Jolly (1918–1986) (Charing Cross Hospital) was appointed as consultant paediatrician to Plymouth in 1951, the Cornish Times with splendid semantic ambiguity commented that the children's feet would now be well cared for. Paterson had to persuade the dubious Still that 'paediatrics' would be spelt with an 'a' before 'the great little man' accepted both the name of the Association and the Presidency.

Still was a bachelor of small physique who always wore a frock coat. He spoke in an unauthoritative low tone of voice but was recognised to have an unrivalled knowledge of childhood disease and of children (as exemplified in the letter to his goddaughter reproduced in Plate 42). He could be impatient with parents but took infinite pains to win over the most refractory child. He was determined that those under his care should suffer least hurt and lumbar punctures and chest tappings usually had to be carried out under his watchful eye. He did regular rounds of his ward at King's College Hospital and on Sunday mornings always made a point of playing with the children, discarding on these occasions the tradition that the ward sister should accompany her 'chief'. He wrote the outstanding 'History of Paediatrics'. Published in 1931, it gave a historical account of the subject from the time of Hippocrates till the end of the eighteenth century [6].

Paterson was the obvious choice as Honorary Secretary of the Association, and Morley Fletcher became Treasurer. The Executive Committee had two members from London, Poynton and Cameron; two from the provinces, Spence and Parsons; and one each from Scotland, Dr T Y (Tiff) Finlay (1882–1953) (Edinburgh), and Northern Ireland, Dr (later Professor) F M B (Freddie) Allen (1898–1972) (Belfast). Of those who were invited to join the new Association, 56 were accepted; 3 others distinguished in the field of medicine were invited to become Honorary Members, namely, Sir Thomas Barlow, Professor Sir Archibald Garrod (1857–1936) and Sir Humphrey Rolleston.

Following its foundation, the growth in membership and influence of the BPA was steady. In the early years, most BPA members were concerned with disease in children occurring beyond the neonatal period. The latter was tradi-tionally an obstetric province, but soon some paediatricians began to extend their interest to the newborn too. That the BPA and its members were slowly being accepted as 'baby' experts was demonstrated by a request in 1936 from Queen Charlotte's Maternity Hospital in London for an answer to the controver-sial problem of 'the standard weight to be accepted for the definition of prema-turity'. Capon and Dr (later Professor Sir Alan) Moncrieff (1901–1971) (Middlesex, GOS and Queen Charlotte's Maternity Hospital) reported the BPA's definition of 5.5 lb (2.5 kg) or less and solved the problem, at least for the time being.

In his history of the early years of the BPA, Cameron wrote with pride of the achievement of the Association in increasing recognition by the then Ministry of Health of the importance of paediatrics as a specialty in its own right. With a vision beyond that of Lord Beveridge in his classic report 'Social Insurance and Allied Services' (1942), Cameron wrote that no limit could be set to the rising cost of treat-ment in hospital under a state health service and went on to argue that better preven-tion of illness and promotion of child health would 'help to make the children of the nation vigorous and strong'.

The Second World War (1939–1945)

With the outbreak of the Second World War, the activities of the Association, par-ticularly its Executive Committee, increased dramatically due to its involvement in safeguarding the health of a child population undergoing mass evacuation. The main burden of all this work fell on the shoulders of Paterson and Moncrieff who worked incessantly during these years. Cameron records the Executive Committee's exertions to mitigate the effect on children of evacuation from our cities, including a plea for the appointment of more paediatricians to look after them. Air raids caused considerable destruction of homes and consequent disruption of family life, but happily plans to deal with vast numbers of displaced and homeless children were not needed.

The Association at this time of stress was fortunate in its leadership. In the turmoil produced by the war, paediatricians such as Parsons, Spence and Professor Charles McNeil (1881–1964) of Edinburgh found full opportunity for the exercise of their powers of organisation, constructive criticism and forward vision. All three held newly established Chairs of Child Health in their universities and were constantly occupied in work on government and other committees of importance. The Executive Committee's work entailed long and tedious railway journeys at a time of great difficulty and even danger because of air raids. Members often arrived for meetings at Paterson's hospitable fireside worn out and exhausted, but he was always the eager host who would house and, despite food rationing, feed them.

A plea by the Association at this time, which has its echoes today, concerned the retention of children's trained nurses in children's wards and children's hospitals. As has happened so many times since, the abolition of the register of sick children's nurses was being mooted. Other subjects of BPA advocacy were the admission of mothers with their children when the latter were admitted to the hospital, the separation of short-stay from long-stay admissions and the provision of education for children in the hospital. Over 40 years later, these practices are still not always observed even though the principles on which they are based are now agreed.

Despite the war, Annual Meetings continued. In 1943 there was a discussion, the first of many, on a proposed College of Child Health. Later in 1943 and in 1944, BPA reports were issued on 'The Organisation of a Paediatric Service', 'Tuberculosis', and 'Rickets'. Medical politics also entered the scene for the first time with the proposed introduction of a National Health Service. At first a medico-political role was unwelcome to many BPA members as it was feared that to meddle in medical politics might cause dissension among paediatricians. There is very little evidence that this happened then or has happened since. Increasingly the Executive Committee received requests for advice about developing the paediatric service. As the war approached its end, there were increasing signs of a new dawn in the field of child health. The 1945 meeting was acknowledged as 'the most successful of all those held under the shadow of the war', probably for two reasons. A victorious peace was imminent, and the meeting was held at Rugby School in the new sanatorium where Dr R E Smith (1901–1983) had established a reputation as a forward-looking school medical officer. He had been elected a member of the BPA in 1939 and was made an Honorary Member 'for wise counsel' in 1969. Many pre-war members of the BPA and a very much larger number of more recent medical graduates destined later to become paediatricians, and members of the BPA served with distinction in the Armed Forces during the war in all parts of the world. Dr Cicely Williams (later Commander of the Order of St Michael and St George), an international figure, and Dr Patrick McArthur (1912–1984) (Inverness) suffered immense privation as prisoners of war each performing outstanding work in the medical care of those, like themselves, incarcerated in prisoner of war and internment camps in the Far East.

The Establishment of University Departments of Child Health

The BPA has been so closely involved with the establishment of university departments of paediatrics and child health that a consideration of their development is a necessary part of the history of the BPA. Some were established before the Second World War, but the war gave an impetus to this academic development. The early university chairs mostly owed their creation to paediatricians of drive and energy whose work was recognised in this manner. A Chair of Medical Diseases of Children was established in Glasgow in 1924 and a Chair of Paediatrics in Birmingham in 1929 due to the influence of Findlay and Parsons, respectively.

The early paediatricians, academic and nonacademic, were concerned primarily with disease. Their wards were full to overflowing with seriously ill children. As children were not covered by the National Health Insurance Act, the hospital paediatric outpatient department was their main source of medical advice, care and treatment in the 1930s. Medical crises were the hospital norm and such paediatricians as there were had to devote their time and energy to dealing with these. Most children, however, are born healthy, and the preservation of their health is as important as, if not more important than, curing established disease. The concept of child health, concerned not just with disease but with the preventive, social and developmental aspects of child health, was developed by McNeil in Edinburgh where in 1931 the first chair embodying these principles, the Chair of Child Life and Health, was established. McNeil was a quiet visionary whose ideas on the importance of developmental paediatrics, community care and neonatal care were ahead of his time.

A revealing story about McNeil was recently recounted by a very elderly retired family practitioner in the Scottish Highlands who, as an undergraduate, had been a medical student in Edinburgh. On a cold winter day early in the 1920s, he was one of a group of students who arrived for the first time at McNeil's ward in the Royal Hospital for Sick Children in Edinburgh to begin his paediatric clinical teaching. The students were met by McNeil who told them to warm their hands at the coal-fired stove which then occupied the centre of the ward. McNeil then left the ward. As the students waited round the stove for his return, they were joined by the more mobile children in the ward, seeking the warmer area round the stove for their play. Students and children were soon talking and even playing together, and it was not long before the children confined to bed were participating in the discourse and commenting freely on the play. The students were relaxed but somewhat mystified at the continued absence of McNeil. An hour and a half later, he reappeared, looked at them with benign approval and announced that the teaching session was now over: he was satisfied that the students had learned the first lesson in paediatrics – how to relate to children.

Spence and Parsons continued McNeil's philosophy. Spence, on his appointment to the Newcastle Chair of Child Health in 1942, wrote to McNeil acknowledging him as the prime originator of the child health concept. He also responded to the congratulations of the BPA in these terms: 'Had it not been for the BPA, I would not have endured in the field of medicine and there would have been no Chair of Child Health or Paediatric Child Medicine, or whatever we decide to call it'. Of Spence's contribution to the child health concept, Cameron wrote: 'Spence, perhaps more than any other of his day, was to join with Parsons in developing that approach to the subject which was envisaged when all the new Professorships in Paediatrics were given the title of Chair of Child Health. With his charming crooked smile and diffident air, he would seem to take his audience into his confidence as he elaborated his argument or set before them a prophetic vision of some new Jerusalem, a vision however that was always based upon months or years of hard thinking and patient investigation'. By the late 1940s and early 1950s, most universities with medical schools, apart from London, had established Chairs of Child Health, a process which was continued later by the establishment of several Chairs of Paediatrics or Child Health in London, Oxford (1972) and Cambridge (1979).

In 1942 English provincial universities' spending on paediatric teaching and research ranged from £20 a year in Sheffield to £90 a year in Bristol. Even in Birmingham, it was only £56 a year. In London, it was approximately £116 for each teaching hospital. The Scots' alleged traditional parsimony certainly did not extend to paediatrics, for the universities of both Edinburgh and Glasgow each allocated to their well-established departments of paediatrics about £2500 a year. The Goodenough Report (1944) recommended that every medical school in Britain should be under the control of a university, and as a result, the financial resources of the universities were greatly increased to meet this responsibility. Extensions and improvements of clinical academic departments became possible, and whole-time clinical professorships and lectureships were established. Spence argued for the establishment of comprehensive university paediatric hospital departments with not less than a hundred beds either in general hospitals or preferably in a children's hospital.

Post-war (1945–1968)

By 1945 there had been little change in the pattern of medical practice. Early parenthood still remained a time of relative penury for many. Young paediatricians, whatever their promise or ability, could not earn sufficient if they confined themselves to paediatric practice. There were still few paediatricians in London and even fewer in the provinces. Fortunately, the NHS, which started on 5th July 1948, changed that and represented a great stride forward in the care of children. Consultants were now paid for their hospital work, and it was possible to develop a service based on consultant paediatricians in every region of the country. Coincidentally the BPA urged, unsuccessfully at that time, that what today are called community child health staff and were then local authority medical staff working in child welfare and school clinics should no longer work in isolation but should be associated with the hospital service. Waller, for instance, whose memorable work on breastfeeding was referred to earlier, served in a local authority infant welfare clinic as well as at the Babies Hospital, Woolwich.

In 1946, at the conclusion of his extended 3-year term of office as President of the BPA, Parsons had been knighted. He had guided the BPA through difficult war years. 1947 had seen the return of the BPA meetings to their original annual meeting place at Windermere, and appropriately Paterson, the virtual founder of the BPA, was President. The following year, he departed for his native Canada as the idea of a National Health Service did not appeal to him.

In 1951, Spence, newly knighted, was President. Parsons had just died, and a fund in his memory was used to provide a President's badge of office and the two silver candlesticks – sadly subsequently stolen – that used to grace the table at the Annual Dinner. In the same year, Sir Robert Hutchison achieved his eightieth birthday. 'Witty and wise, able to guide discussion along lines of reason and common sense, he was held in esteem by all members for his clinical wisdom and for encouraging anything promising but preserving a chilling douche for whatever was extravagant, pretentious or over-enthusiastic'. It is recorded that at one BPA meeting, where a speaker had given a preliminary communication quite inadequate in content and logic, Sir Robert rose and, elongating himself to his full 6 feet 3 inches, addressed the speaker thus, 'I observe that you have entitled your paper a preliminary communication. I think that you would be well advised to make it also a final communication'. He was one of the great teachers of paediatrics of the past, and his 'Lectures on Diseases of Children' [7] was owned by almost every senior BPA member.

Although obstetricians had traditionally cared for the newborn and had often opposed any proposal that paediatricians should be involved to any major extent in neonatal care, some obstetricians were now inviting paediatricians to enter the erstwhile secret realm of the labour room in addition to their responsibilities in the neonatal nursery. Gradually total care of the newborn became an increasing responsibility and preoccupation of paediatricians. Imagine a newborn unit now without a paediatrician in charge!

After existing for nearly 25 years, the Association had gained in influence and importance. It was strong enough to confront the Ministry of Health and had occasion to do so. The Ministry had proposed a reduction in the number of senior registrars. The arguments against this proposal were a little different from those of today and no less convincing. Were not children surviving and requiring medical attention where formerly they had died? Had not new diseases been recognised to justify the need for more rather than fewer trainees? Renal acidosis, toxoplasmosis, cystic fibrosis, retrolental fibroplasia and subdural haematoma had all been described in recent years. The Ministry had taken no account of the advances in, and widening scope of, paediatrics and the need to match these developments by the appointment of more consultants.

Much of the emphasis in the 1950s was falling on the development of regional paediatric services, and in conjunction with this, Regional Paediatric Societies were established in England and Wales. At the Annual Meeting of the BPA in 1959, the evening session was devoted to 'The Problems of the Regional Paediatrician'. Most regional paediatricians were working single handed in isolation dealing with populations in areas so large that many hours were spent travelling. Colleagues were needed urgently. The BPA now assembled the requirements for a properly staffed comprehensive national paediatric service.

During these years, the organisation of comprehensive children's hospitals and children's departments in general hospitals was the subject of much discussion. The BPA continued to stress the need for children's hospitals or adequate children's wards and separate outpatient and casualty departments for children. Surgeons, radiologists and pathologists trained to deal with children and children's diseases were required. In 1954 the British Association of Paediatric Surgeons was founded. The BPA was also working to bring the wards occupied by children and beds for children in infectious disease hospitals under the general care of paediatricians. Paediatricians were responsible for only a quarter of all beds for children in infectious disease hospitals. Some of these once busy hospitals, with their cubicles, masked and gowned staff and smell of carbolic, were now less necessary and less relevant. They were separated from general hospitals, often by many miles, had separate staff and in some instances had not kept pace with the burgeoning knowledge of paediatrics. The BPA also sought closer cooperation with Medical Officers of Health and general practitioners, a harder task in the climate of the 1950s than it would be today, for the Association's advice was often ignored.

As serious and fatal childhood disease diminished, important psychological problems associated with the hospitalisation of children became better recognised and were a challenge to nursing and paediatric practice. The rigid rule that children in hospital should be visited for 2 h on Sundays only, visits ending so often with the screams of the children and the weeping of parents, was recognised as a serious neglect of children's needs. Some hospitals not only allowed visiting but began to encourage it. Mothers – and even fathers – were invited to stay with their children. Spence at the Mother and Babies Hospital in Newcastle was one of the chief protagonists of these developments. Later, in 1966, the Minister of Health accepted the recommendation of the Platt Report (1959) (Sir Harry Platt, an Honorary Member of the BPA, died in his 101st year in 1986) on the 'Welfare of Children in Hospital' [8] that 'unrestricted' visiting and admission of mothers with their children should be implemented. This was hardly achieved overnight. In some areas, nurses, administrators and doctors more attuned to the needs of adults than children took years to become converted. Of great help was the establishment in 1961 of the National Association for the Welfare of Children in Hospital (NAWCH). The problem is not yet solved. Even in 1987, a survey, 'Where Are the Children?' [9], in which NAWCH and the BPA participated, showed that a quarter of the children in hospital were still being cared for in wards for adults. Equally revolutionary was the move to allow children to retain their own clothes and possessions while in hospital! These and many other changes were vigorously promoted by the BPA.

In 1965 Paterson wrote to a young paediatrician, 'Watch where paediatrics is going and prepare for it. In 1920 we approached a sick child armed with a stethoscope and a few drugs - mastoiditis, meningitis, pneumonia seemed often beyond help. Now we have entered another phase, the war on genetic disease, congenital malformations including damage in utero to the unborn infant from maternal infections, toxic action of drugs, poor nutrition and lack of oxygen; the age of preventive paediatrics is upon us and early diagnosis and early treatment are parts of prevention'. In 1968 Neale commented in his history: '... cytogenetics must now be included in concepts of aetiology'. Chromosome identification followed by major advances in the understanding of genetic disease was constituting one of the great advances in paediatrics comparable to the advent of radiology in diagnosis and antibiotics in the treatment of infection.

In the field of education, the BPA Education Committee's report on 'Careers in Paediatrics' stressed the significance of clinical, family and community work in the care of children. Of community care of children, Neale wrote: 'No branch of medicine has advanced more rapidly or widened its scope so much'. How pleased he would have been to see the progressive and necessary expansion of the community child health services and the gradual abandonment of the barriers which had existed between paediatricians working in the hospital service and the then Medical Officers of Health and their clinical counterparts working in the community child health service.

The BPA's primary purpose of advancing the cause of children and promoting child health was gaining momentum and with this came greater respect and recognition for the subject. There was still a long way to go, however. The paediatric and child health service was incomplete and fragmented; many aspects of paediatric training were unsatisfactory; health authorities, universities and government still needed much persuasion and constant prompting.

References

1. Neale AV. The British Paediatric Association 1952-1968. London: Pitman; 1970.
2. Thomas Phaire. 'The Boke of Chyldren'. 1544. Republished 1955 (Neale, A.V. and Wallis, H.R.E.). E & S Livingstone. Edinburgh and London.
3. Maloney WJ. George and John Armstrong of Castleton. Edinburgh: E & S Livingstone; 1954.
4. Armstrong G. An essay on the diseases most fatal to infants. London: Cadell T; 1767.
5. Cameron HC. The nervous child. London: Henry Frowde, Hodder and Stoughton; 1919.
6. Still GF. The history of paediatrics. Oxford and London: Oxford University Press; 1931.
7. Hutchison R. Lectures on diseases of children. London: Edward Arnold; 1904.
8. Ministry of Health. The welfare of children in hospital. London: HMSO; 1958.
9. National Association for the Welfare of Children in Hospital. Where are the Children? UK: Cheadle Hulme; 1987.

Senior Officers of BPA and RCPCH

President	
1985–1988	Professor John Forfar
1988–1991	Professor Dame June Lloyd
1991–1994	Professor Sir David Hull
1994–1997	Professor Sir Roy Meadow
1997–1999	Professor David Baum
1999–2000	Professor Richard Cooke
2000–2003	Professor Sir David Hall
2003–2006	Professor Sir Alan Craft
2006–2009	Dr Patricia Hamilton
2009–2012	Professor Terence Stephenson
2012–2015	Dr Hilary Cass
2015 –	Professor Neena Modi

Honorary Secretary/Registrar	
1984–1989	Dr Tim Chambers
1989–1994	Dr Roddie McFaul
1994–1999	Dr Keith Dodd
1999–2003	Dr Patricia Hamilton
2003–2006	Dr Sheila Shribman
2006–2008	Dr Hilary Cass
2008–2011	Dr David Vickers
2011–2012	Professor Hamish Wallace
2012 –	Dr Ian Maconochie